Imaging of the Aorta

Iacopo Carbone · Davide Farina
Pier Giorgio Nardis · Davide Bellini
Editors

Imaging of the Aorta

A Practical Guide for Radiologists

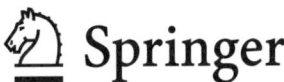

Editors
Iacopo Carbone
Academic Diagnostic Imaging Division
Department of Medical-Surgical Sciences
and Biotechnologies
Faculty of Pharmacy and Medicine
I.C.O.T. Hospital
University of Rome "Sapienza"
Latina, LT, Italy

Pier Giorgio Nardis
Vascular and Interventional Radiology
Sapienza University of Rome
Rome, Italy

Davide Farina
Department of Radiology
University of Brescia
Brescia, Italy

Davide Bellini
Academic Diagnostic Imaging Division
Sapienza University of Rome
Latina, Italy

ISBN 978-3-031-52529-2   ISBN 978-3-031-52527-8 (eBook)
https://doi.org/10.1007/978-3-031-52527-8

Translation from the Italian language edition: "Imaging aortico" by Iacopo Carbone et al., © Copyright © 2021 Davide Bellini, Iacopo Carbone, Davide Farina, Pier Giorgio Nardis 2021. Published by n/a. All Rights Reserved.

The translation was done with the help of an artificial intelligence machine translation tool. A subsequent human revision was done primarily in terms of content.

© The Editor(s) (if applicable) and The Author(s), under exclusive license to Springer Nature Switzerland AG 2024

This work is subject to copyright. All rights are solely and exclusively licensed by the Publisher, whether the whole or part of the material is concerned, specifically the rights of reprinting, reuse of illustrations, recitation, broadcasting, reproduction on microfilms or in any other physical way, and transmission or information storage and retrieval, electronic adaptation, computer software, or by similar or dissimilar methodology now known or hereafter developed.

The use of general descriptive names, registered names, trademarks, service marks, etc. in this publication does not imply, even in the absence of a specific statement, that such names are exempt from the relevant protective laws and regulations and therefore free for general use.

The publisher, the authors and the editors are safe to assume that the advice and information in this book are believed to be true and accurate at the date of publication. Neither the publisher nor the authors or the editors give a warranty, expressed or implied, with respect to the material contained herein or for any errors or omissions that may have been made. The publisher remains neutral with regard to jurisdictional claims in published maps and institutional affiliations.

This Springer imprint is published by the registered company Springer Nature Switzerland AG
The registered company address is: Gewerbestrasse 11, 6330 Cham, Switzerland

If disposing of this product, please recycle the paper.

To Marina, my beloved friend
—Iacopo

Foreword

A man [...] was seized with a pain of the right arm and soon after of the left, [...] after these there appeared a tumor on the upper part of the sternum [...] He was ordered to think seriously and piously of his departure from this mortal life, which was very near at hand and inevitable. (G B Morgagni, from: M. Klompas: JAMA. 2002, 287, S. 2262–2272)

This is one of the first (or maybe the first!) descriptions of an acute aortic syndrome that can be found in literature. And how amazing to see what has become possible in aortic medicine thanks to the interaction of improved diagnostic and therapeutic possibilities! Aortic diseases remain life-threatening by nature, but they don't describe necessarily the end of life anymore! Despite the importance of aortic diseases—it's about THE main artery!—and the exciting evolution in diagnosis and therapy, comprehensive books dedicated to aortic imaging are rare.

Iacopo Carbone, a well-known expert in cardiovascular radiology, and his coauthors, representing a carefully selected group of experts, succeed in their attempts to fill this gap. They provide us with a state-of-the-art compilation of all-you-need-to-know about imaging on aortic diseases. A special focus is addressed to the imaging follow-up after therapy, representing a growing field of application of aortic radiology. An additional fantastic feature of this exciting book is the reporting checklist at the end of most of the chapters, representing a very practical tool to avoid common mistakes.

I can just congratulate the team around Iacopo Carbone for their efforts in putting together this fantastic book filling a real need and representing an indispensable resource for modern aortic radiology. I wish the readers of this volume a lot of fun and exciting insights into the fascinating field of aortic radiology.

Division of Cardiovascular
and Interventional Radiology,
Department for Bioimaging
and Image-Guided Therapy
Medical University of Vienna,
Vienna, Austria

Christian Loewe

Preface

The aorta is under the eyes of any general radiologist almost every day, either because its assessment is the primary goal of an exam or simply because it is included in the field of view.

In some cases, the clinical scenario makes the interpretation of images straightforward; in other cases, significant pathologic findings might be without symptoms and are detected incidentally. The ability to differentiate minor from relevant findings, even more so when these are subtle, is therefore necessary.

In addition, not infrequently, the severity of the clinical presentation demands a significant acceleration of the work of the radiologist. Not only the interpretation must be correct, but the report must also be produced in a very short time and must go straight to the point, conveying the clinically relevant findings in few precise words.

This manual gathers the long-standing professional experience of a group of radiologists and friends. The aim that inspired us was to support younger radiologists in these routine tasks, providing a succinct description of relevant clinical and imaging findings and guiding their reporting with essential checklists.

Latina, Italy	Iacopo Carbone
Brescia, Italy	Davide Farina
Rome, Italy	Pier Giorgio Nardis
Latina, Italy	Davide Bellini

Contents

Part I Anatomy and Imaging Techniques

1. **Anatomy and Standardized Terminology**................. 3
   Davide Bellini and Antonio Capodanno

2. **Aortic Study Technique: Angio-TC: Minimum Criteria and State of the Art**................................ 15
   Federica Giulio, Nicola Panvini, and Marco Rengo

3. **MR-Angiography: Basic and Optional Sequences**................. 21
   Placido Romeo, Antonio Celona, and Maria Cristina Inserra

4. **Transthoracic and Transesophageal Echocardiography**........... 29
   Elena Cavarretta

5. **Ultrasound of the Abdominal Aorta** 35
   Simone Vicini, Paola Lucchesi, Marco Maria Maceroni, and Elena Orlando

Part II The Aorta on the Chest X-Ray

6. **Anatomical Landmarks: Lines and Stripes** 41
   Maria Dea Ippoliti, Emanuela Algeri, and Iacopo Carbone

7. **Abnormal Findings**.. 45
   Maria Dea Ippoliti, Emanuela Algeri, and Iacopo Carbone

Part III Aortic Aneurysms: Pre-treatment Evaluation

8. **Thoracic Aortic Diseases** 53
   Pier Giorgio Nardis, Bianca Rocco, Simone Ciaglia, Mario Corona, Simone Zilahi de Gyurgyokai, and Carlo Catalano

9. **Thoracoabdominal Aortic Aneurysm (Classification, CT Aspects, Pre-Procedure Evaluation, Endovascular Treatment)** 69
   Ciro Ferrer

10 **Abdominal Aortic Aneurysm** 83
    Pier Giorgio Nardis, Simone Ciaglia, Bianca Rocco,
    Simone Zilahi de Gyurgyokai, Alessandro Cannavale,
    and Carlo Catalano

11 **Aortic Aneurysm in Emergency: Radiological Signs
    of Pre-Rupture and of Rupture** 103
    Nicolò Schicchi, Leonardo Teodoli, Pierleone Lucatelli,
    Paolo Esposto Pirani, Marco Fogante, Fatjon Cela,
    and Liliana Balardi

12 **Reporting Checklist: Endovascular Pre-Treatment** 111
    Bianca Rocco, Simone Ciaglia, Pierleone Lucatelli, Carlo Catalano,
    and Pier Giorgio Nardis

Part IV Aortic Aneurysms: Follow-Up

13 **Follow-Up After Endovascular Aneurysm Repair** 117
    Valentina Chiara Romano

14 **Follow-Up of Untreated Aneurysm** 125
    Angelo Iannarelli and Giovanni Trillò

15 **Reporting Checklist: Aneurysm Follow-Up
    of the Abdominal Aorta** 131
    Angelo Iannarelli, Giovanni Trillò, and Valentina Romano

Part V Acute Aortic Syndrome

16 **Acute Aortic Syndrome (AAS) and Traumatic Aortic
    Injury (TAI)** 135
    Filippo Vaccher, Davide Farina, Andrea Borghesi,
    and Marco Ravanelli

17 **Aortic Dissection: Imaging and Elements of Endovascular
    Pretreatment Evaluation** 151
    Nicolò Schicchi, Matteo Marcucci, Paolo Esposto Pirani,
    Marco Fogante, Fatjon Cela, and Liliana Balardi

18 **Reporting Checklist: Acute Aortic Syndromes** 163
    Filippo Vaccher

Part VI Inflammatory Diseases of the Aorta

19 **Imaging Methods: General Principles** 167
    Filippo Vaccher, Davide Farina, Emanuela Algeri,
    and Marco Ravanelli

20	**Giant Cell Arteritis, Takayasu Arteritis, Chronic Periaortitis, Infectious Aortitis**.............................	171
	Filippo Vaccher, Davide Farina, Emanuela Algeri, and Marco Ravanelli	
21	**Reporting Checklist: Inflammatory Diseases of the Aorta**..........	181
	Filippo Vaccher, Davide Farina, Emanuela Algeri, and Marco Ravanelli	

Part VII Congenital Anomalies of the Thoracic Aorta: An Overview

22	**Aortic Dilatation and Aortopathies in Congenital Heart Disease**...	185
	Paolo Ciancarella, Veronica Bordonaro, and Aurelio Secinaro	
23	**Congenital Obstructive Heart Disease**	191
	Paolo Ciancarella, Veronica Bordonaro, and Aurelio Secinaro	
24	**Anatomical Variants and Congenital Anomalies of the Aortic Arch**	197
	Paolo Ciancarella, Veronica Bordonaro, and Aurelio Secinaro	

Part VIII Taking It to the Test

25	**Clinical Cases**	209
	Federica Giulio, Elena Orlando, Alessandro Onori, Simone Ciaglia, Bianca Rocco, Pier Giorgio Nardis, Davide Curione, Nunzia Di Meo, and Teresa Falcone	

Contributors

Emanuela Algeri Service de Radiologie et Imagerie Cardiovasculaire, Hôpital Cardiologique, Centre Hospitalier Régional et Universitaire de Lille, Lille Cedex, France

Liliana Balardi Azienda Ospedaliero Universitaria "Ospedali Riuniti", Ancona, Italy

Davide Bellini Academic Diagnostic Imaging Division, Department of Medical-Surgical Sciences and Biotechnologies, Faculty of Pharmacy and Medicine, I.C.O.T. Hospital, "Sapienza" University of Rome, Latina, LT, Italy

Veronica Bordonaro Department of Imaging, Advanced Cardiovascular Imaging Unit, Bambino Gesù Children's Hospital, IRCCS, Rome, Italy

Advanced Cardiothoracic Imaging Unit, Bambino Gesù Children's Hospital, IRCCS, Rome, Italy

Andrea Borghesi Institute of Radiology, Department of Medical and Surgical Specialties, Radiological Sciences, and Public Health, University of Brescia, Brescia, Italy

Alessandro Cannavale Vascular and Interventional Radiology Unit, Department of Radiological, Oncological and Anathomo-Pathological Science, Policlinico Umberto I, "Sapienza" University of Rome, Rome, Italy

Antonio Capodanno Academic Diagnostic Imaging Division, Department of Medical-Surgical Sciences and Biotechnologies, Faculty of Pharmacy and Medicine, I.C.O.T. Hospital, "Sapienza" University of Rome, Latina, LT, Italy

Iacopo Carbone Academic Diagnostic Imaging Division, Department of Medical-Surgical Sciences and Biotechnologies, Faculty of Pharmacy and Medicine, I.C.O.T. Hospital, University of Rome "Sapienza", Latina, LT, Italy

Carlo Catalano Vascular and Interventional Radiology Unit, Department of Radiological, Oncological and Anathomo-patological Science, Policlinico Umberto I, "Sapienza" University of Rome, Rome, Italy

Elena Cavarretta Department of Medical-Surgical Sciences and Biotechnologies, Sapienza University of Rome, Latina, Italy

Fatjon Cela SOD Materno-Infantile, Cardiologica, Senologica ed Ecografia Ambulatoriale, Azienda Ospedaliero Universitaria "Ospedali Riuniti", Ancona, Italy

Antonio Celona UOC Radiologia, AO Papardo, Messina, Italy

Simone Ciaglia Vascular and Interventional Radiology Unit, Department of Radiological, Oncological and Anathomo-patological Science, Policlinico Umberto I, "Sapienza" University of Rome, Rome, Italy

Paolo Ciancarella Department of Imaging, Advanced Cardiovascular Imaging Unit, Bambino Gesù Children's Hospital, IRCCS, Rome, Italy

Advanced Cardiothoracic Imaging Unit, Bambino Gesù Children's Hospital, IRCCS, Rome, Italy

Mario Corona Vascular and Interventional Radiology Unit, Department of Radiological, Oncological and Anathomo-patological Science, Policlinico Umberto I, "Sapienza" University of Rome, Rome, Italy

Davide Curione Advanced Cardiovascular Imaging Unit, Department of Imaging, Bambino Gesù Children's Hospital, IRCCS, Rome, Italy

Simone Zilahi de Gyurgyokai Vascular and Interventional Radiology Unit, Department of Radiological, Oncological and Anathomo-patological Science, Policlinico Umberto I, "Sapienza" University of Rome, Rome, Italy

Nunzia Di Meo Department of Medical and Surgical Specialties, Radiological Sciences, and Public Health, University of Brescia, Brescia, Italy

Radiology Unit 2, ASST Spedali Civili di Brescia, Brescia, Italy

Teresa Falcone Department of Medical and Surgical Specialties, Radiological Sciences, and Public Health, University of Brescia, Brescia, Italy

Radiology Unit 2, ASST Spedali Civili di Brescia, Brescia, Italy

Davide Farina Institute of Radiology, Department of Medical and Surgical Specialties, Radiological Sciences, and Public Health, University of Brescia, Brescia, Italy

Radiology Unit 2, ASST Spedali Civili di Brescia, Brescia, Italy

Ciro Ferrer Vascular and Endovascular Surgery Unit, San Giovanni-Addolorata Hospital, Rome, Italy

Marco Fogante SOD Materno-Infantile, Cardiologica, Senologica ed Ecografia Ambulatoriale, Azienda Ospedaliero Universitaria "Ospedali Riuniti", Ancona, Italy

Federica Giulio Department of Radiological, Oncological and Pathological Sciences, "Sapienza" University of Rome, I.C.O.T. Hospital, Latina, LT, Italy

Angelo Iannarelli Department of Diagnostic and Interventional Radiology, Santa Maria Goretti Hospital, Latina, Italy

Maria Cristina Inserra UOSD Radiologia CAST, AOU Policlinico "G. Rodolico", San Marco, Catania, Italy

Maria Dea Ippoliti Department of Radiological, Oncological and Pathological Sciences, "Sapienza" University of Rome, I.C.O.T. Hospital, Latina, LT, Italy

Pierleone Lucatelli Interventional Radiology Section of Department of Radiological, Oncological, and Anatomopathological, Sciences of Policlinico Umberto I of Rome, Sapienza University of Rome, Rome, Italy

Paola Lucchesi Department of Radiological, Oncological and Pathological Sciences, "Sapienza" University of Rome, I.C.O.T. Hospital, Latina, LT, Italy

Marco Maria Maceroni Department of Radiological, Oncological and Pathological Sciences, "Sapienza" University of Rome, I.C.O.T. Hospital, Latina, LT, Italy

Matteo Marcucci U.O.C. di Radiodiagnostica, Ospedale Generale Provinciale di Macerata, Macerata, Italy

Pier Giorgio Nardis Vascular and Interventional Radiology Unit, Department of Radiological, Oncological and Anathomo-patological Science, Policlinico Umberto I, "Sapienza" University of Rome, Rome, Italy

Alessandro Onori Academic Diagnostic Imaging Division, Faculty of Pharmacy and Medicine, Department of Medical-Surgical Sciences and Biotechnologies, University of Rome "Sapienza", I.C.O.T. Hospital, Latina, Italy

Elena Orlando Department of Radiological, Oncological and Pathological Sciences, "Sapienza" University of Rome, I.C.O.T. Hospital, Latina, LT, Italy

Nicola Panvini Department of Radiological, Oncological and Pathological Sciences, "Sapienza" University of Rome, I.C.O.T. Hospital, Latina, LT, Italy

Paolo Esposto Pirani SOD di Radiologia Materno-Infantile, Senologica, Cardiologica ed Ecografica Ambulatoriale, Azienda Ospedaliero Universitaria "Ospedali Riuniti", Ancona, Italy

SOD Materno-Infantile, Senologica, Cardiologica ed Ecografica Ambulatoriale, Azienda Ospedaliero Universitaria "Ospedali Riuniti", Ancona, Italy

Marco Ravanelli Institute of Radiology, Department of Medical and Surgical Specialties, Radiological Sciences, and Public Health, University of Brescia, Brescia, Italy

Radiology Unit 2, ASST Spedali Civili di Brescia, Brescia, Italy

Marco Rengo Department of Radiological, Oncological and Pathological Sciences, "Sapienza" University of Rome, I.C.O.T. Hospital, Latina, LT, Italy

Bianca Rocco Vascular and Interventional Radiology Unit, Department of Radiological, Oncological and Anathomo-patological Science, Policlinico Umberto I, "Sapienza" University of Rome, Rome, Italy

Valentina Romano Department of Radiology, Charité Universitaetsmedizin Berlin, Berlin, Germany

Valentina Chiara Romano Department of Radiology, Charité Universitaetsmedizin Berlin, Berlin, Germany

Placido Romeo UOC Radiologia San Marco, AOU Policlinico "G. Rodolico", San Marco, Catania, Italy

Nicolò Schicchi SOS Diagnostica Radiologica Cardiovascolare, Azienda Ospedaliero Universitaria "Ospedali Riuniti", Ancona, Italy

Aurelio Secinaro Department of Imaging, Advanced Cardiovascular Imaging Unit, Bambino Gesù Children's Hospital, IRCCS, Rome, Italy

Advanced Cardiothoracic Imaging Unit, Bambino Gesù Children's Hospital, IRCCS, Rome, Italy

Leonardo Teodoli Interventional Radiology Section of Department of Radiological, Oncological, and Anatomopathological, Sciences of Policlinico Umberto I of Rome, Sapienza University of Rome, Rome, Italy

Giovanni Trillò Department of Diagnostic and Interventional Radiology, Santa Maria Goretti Hospital, Latina, Italy

Filippo Vaccher Institute of Radiology, Department of Medical and Surgical Specialties, Radiological Sciences, and Public Health, University of Brescia, Brescia, Italy

Radiology Unit 1, ASST Spedali Civili di Brescia, Brescia, Italy

Simone Vicini Department of Radiological, Oncological and Pathological Sciences, "Sapienza" University of Rome, I.C.O.T. Hospital, Latina, LT, Italy

Part I

Anatomy and Imaging Techniques

Anatomy and Standardized Terminology

Davide Bellini and Antonio Capodanno

Introduction

The aorta is the main artery of the human body, and it receives blood from the left ventricle and distributes it to the systemic circulation. It has a length of approximately 30–40 cm and a caliber of about 2.5–3.5 cm. It is divided into two main districts: the thoracic aorta and the abdominal aorta (Fig. 1.1).

Like all arterial vessels, it has a wall consisting of three juxtaposed layers (Fig. 1.2), from the lumen outward:

- Inner layer (tunica intima), consisting of endothelium resting on the basal lamina;
- Middle layer (tunica media), consisting of alternating layers of smooth muscle cells and elastic fibers;
- Outer layer (tunica adventitia), consisting of connective tissue and vasa vasorum, the nutritious vessels of the arterial wall.

D. Bellini (✉) · A. Capodanno
Academic Diagnostic Imaging Division, Department of Medical-Surgical Sciences and Biotechnologies, Faculty of Pharmacy and Medicine, I.C.O.T. Hospital, "Sapienza" University of Rome, Latina, LT, Italy
e-mail: davide.bellini@uniroma1.it

© The Author(s), under exclusive license to Springer Nature Switzerland AG 2024
I. Carbone et al. (eds.), *Imaging of the Aorta*,
https://doi.org/10.1007/978-3-031-52527-8_1

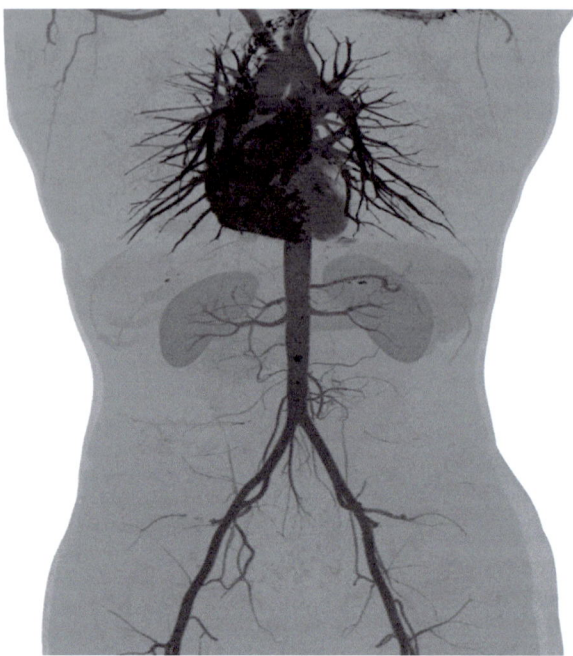

Fig. 1.1 Volume rendering (VR) reconstruction of the entire aorta that resemble angiography

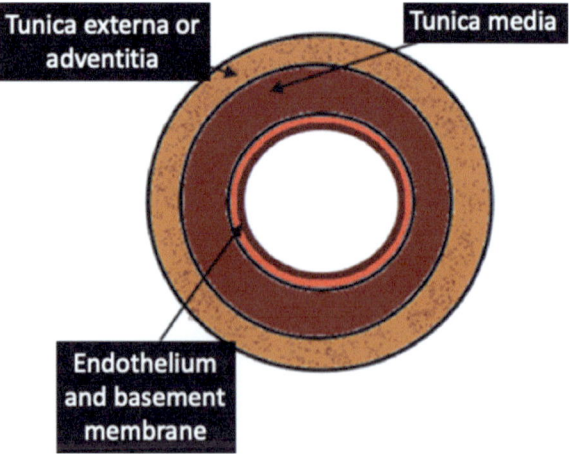

Fig. 1.2 Aortic wall layers

Thoracic Aorta

The thoracic aorta (Fig. 1.3) is located in the thoracic cavity and runs within the mediastinum. It is divided into:

- aortic root;
- ascending aorta;
- aortic arch;
- descending aorta.

Fig. 1.3 Cinematic rendering reconstruction of the thoracic aorta

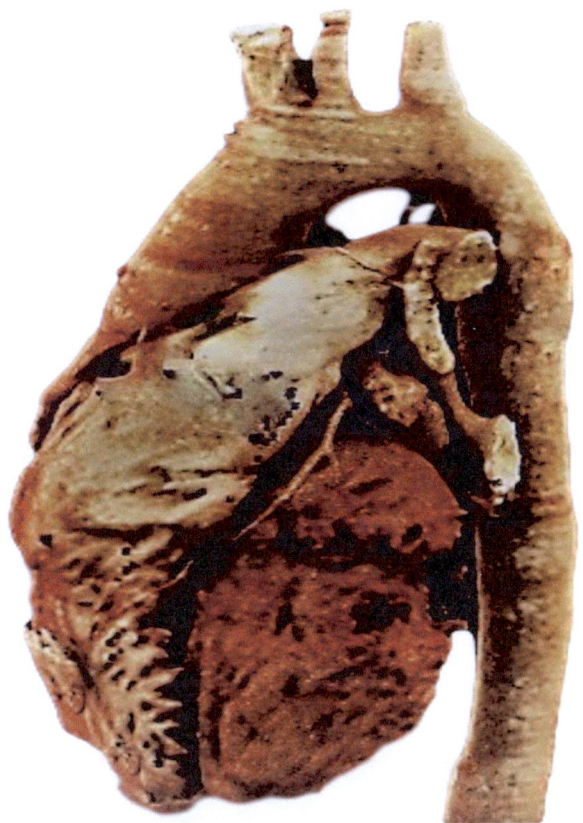

Aortic Root—Ascending Aorta

The root is the most proximal part of the thoracic aorta, extending longitudinally for about 3–4 cm; due to its peculiar globular morphology it is also called aortic bulb. It consists of the semilunar valve and the sinuses of Valsalva, three bulges, two of which (left and right coronary sinuses) give rise to the homonymous coronary arteries; the third sinus is defined non-coronary. The virtual line that joins the insertion points of the three valve leaflets is defined annulus and represents a fundamental landmark for some interventional procedures. It is important to emphasize that the annulus is located upstream of the anatomical junction between the left ventricle and the aorta, therefore in the ventricular cavity (Fig. 1.4).

At the distal end of the sinuses of Valsalva a focal narrowing, the sino-tubular junction, marks the limit between the root and the ascending tubular aorta.

The ascending aorta extends up and to the left to continue, beyond the emergence of the brachiocephalic trunk, into the arch. At the junction with the arch a small dilatation is detectable, the great aortic sinus, a frequent site of aneurysms [1].

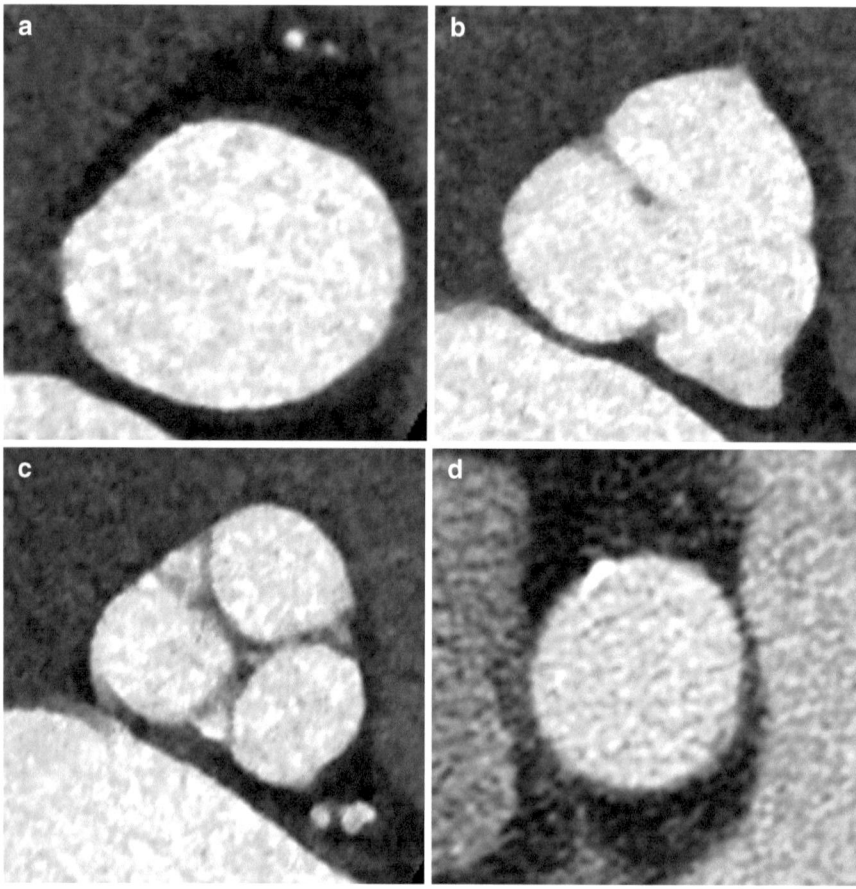

Fig. 1.4 (**a**) The bottom of the aortic root is formed by the virtual ring, or aortic annulus, which is usually oval in shape. (**b**) Ventriculo-valvular junction; leaflets are barely visible at this level. (**c**) The valvular plane: the aortic root assumes a trefoil morphology at the sinuses of Valsalva. On the left, the emergence of the common trunk. (**d**) The sino-tubular junction corresponds to the upper part of the corona, at the transition between the aortic root and ascending aorta

The normal diameter of the root and ascending aorta are extremely variable depending on many factors such as age, sex, and physical constitution (body surface area, BSA). For a practical point of view, normal values are considered: aortic annulus 20–31 mm, sinuses of Valsalva 29–45 mm, sino-tubular junction and ascending aorta 22–36 mm. However, it is advisable, even in daily practice, to refer to normalized values, which are available in the literature (Fig. 1.5) [2, 3].

Fig. 1.5 Aortic root and ascending aorta in the para-coronal MPR plane. Normal reference values, minimum value, maximum value, and "aortic size index" (aortic size/body surface area)

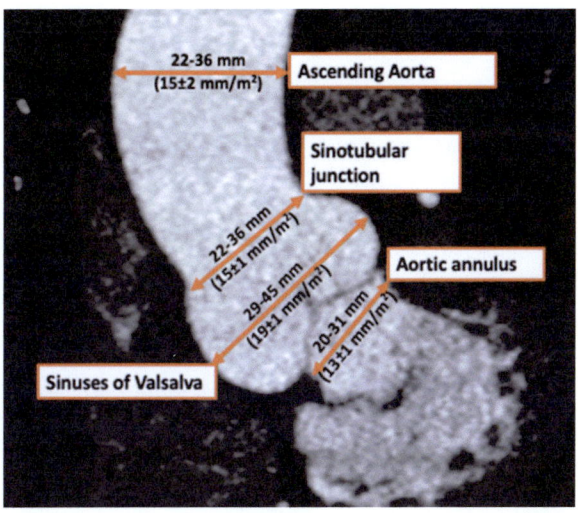

Aortic Arch

This is the segment from which the brachiocephalic trunk (or brachiocephalic artery or innominate artery), the left common carotid artery and the left subclavian artery originate, branches that provide blood supply to the upper limbs and to the head and neck area [4, 5].

It continues the ascending aorta at the level of a plane passing through the manubriosternal joint (Ludwig's plane), it runs from right to left, in an antero-posterior direction, to continue, at the level of a plane corresponding to the IV dorsal vertebra, in the descending aorta. At the transition point between the arch and the descending aorta there is a focal narrowing of the lumen (aortic isthmus), followed by an increase in caliber (aortic spindle). In fetal life, the Botallo's duct, which connects the aorta and the pulmonary artery, is located here; in adult life, occasionally, its vestiges can be seen.

The range of normal diameter values is 22–30 mm.

Collateral Branches of the Aortic Arch

From the convex aspect of the aortic arch originates in sequence the brachiocephalic trunk, the left common carotid artery and the left subclavian artery (the most common morphological pattern, present in about 80% of the population) (Fig. 1.6). In 15% of cases, from the aortic arch originates a large branch called "bovine trunk," from which emerge the brachiocephalic trunk, the right and left common carotid arteries.

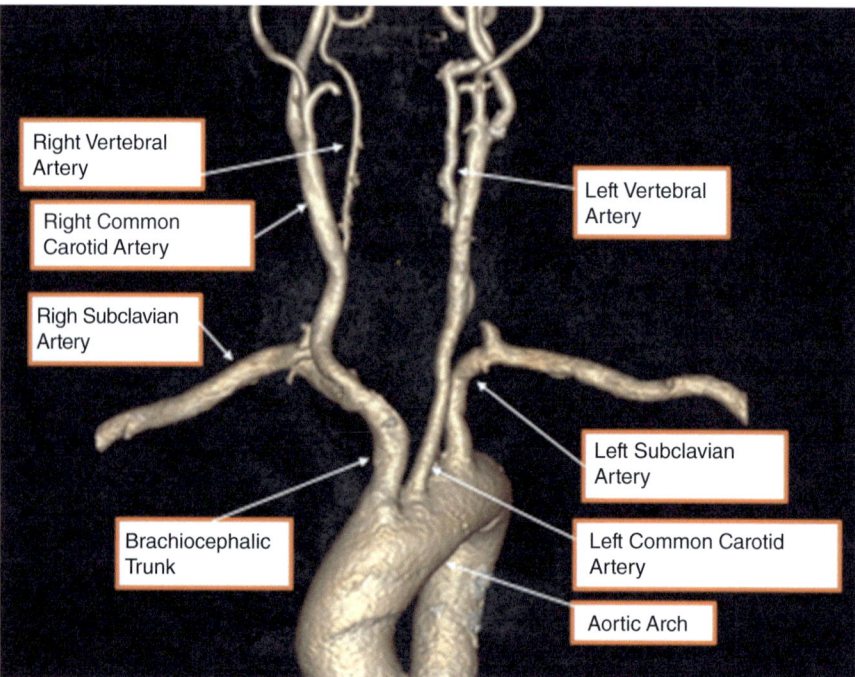

Fig. 1.6 3D Volume rendering reconstruction of the aortic arch and its major branches

Descending Aorta

The descending aorta runs in the posterior mediastinum, from a plane passing through the IV dorsal vertebra to the XII vertebra, where it continues into the abdominal aorta through the aortic hiatus of the diaphragm. It has contiguous relationships with the anterolateral aspect of vertebral bodies, throughout connective septa between the tunica adventitia and the anterior longitudinal ligament. Anteriorly it is related to the left atrium and esophagus. Parietal branches (posterior intercostal, superior phrenic, subcostal) and visceral branches (bronchial, pericardial, mediastinal, and esophageal arteries) originate from the descending aorta [4, 5].

The range of normal diameter values is 22–30 mm.

Pericardial Recesses

The ascending aorta is contained in the fibrous sac of the pericardium and is lined, along with the pulmonary artery, by the visceral leaflet of the pericardium. The visceral pericardium surrounds the heart and the great vessels, forming two main invaginations called sinuses. Posterior to the left atrium, between the superior and inferior vena cava and the four pulmonary veins, there is the oblique pericardial sinus.

Between aorta, pulmonary artery (anteriorly), and atria (posteriorly), we find the transverse pericardial sinus. Within and adjacent to each we can find further inlets called pericardial recesses, often mistakenly identified as lymphadenopathies on computed tomography (CT) examination. From the transverse pericardial sinus originate the superior aortic recess and the inferior aortic recess (aortic recesses) and the right and left pulmonary recesses (pulmonary recesses). We then find the postcaval recess (posterior to the superior vena cava, between the right superior pulmonary vein and right pulmonary artery) and the right and left pulmonary venous recesses.

Abdominal Aorta

The abdominal aorta is the main blood vessel in the abdominal cavity.

It originates at the level of the XII thoracic vertebra and extends up to the level of the IV lumbar vertebra, where it bifurcates into the two common iliac arteries (Fig. 1.7).

Relationship:

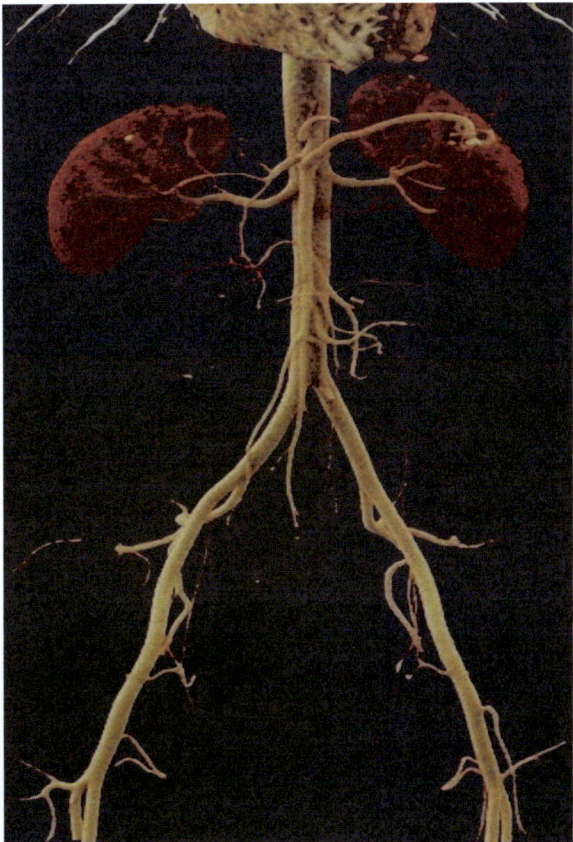

Fig. 1.7 3D Volume rendering reconstruction of the abdominal aorta

- Posteriorly, it is attached to the vertebral soma, running to the left in the initial tract, on the median line in the more caudal portions; it is contiguous to the thoracic duct and to the left lumbar veins;
- Anteriorly, it is surrounded by the celiac and aortic nerve plexuses; it contracts relations with duodenum, pancreas, mesentery, lienal vein, and left renal vein;
- On the right. it is contiguous with inferior vena cava, middle pillar of the diaphragm, caudate lobe of the liver, azygos vein and thoracic duct;
- On the left, it is contiguous with the adrenal gland, renal pelvis, left ureter, and left psoas muscle.

It has single and even branches.

Collateral Branches of the Abdominal Aorta

Single Branches
Celiac tripod, also known as Haller's celiac tripod, arises on the anterior wall of the aorta at the level of the 12th dorsal vertebra. It gives rise to the splenic artery, the left gastric artery, and the gastrohepatic artery (Fig. 1.8) [6, 7].

Splenic artery: it has a tortuous course; it is located retroperitoneally posterior to the stomach, runs along the superior margin of the pancreas. It gives rise to pancreatic branches, short gastric arteries, and lienal branches; caudally it gives rise to the left gastroepiploic artery which anastomoses with the right gastroepiploic artery.

Left gastric artery: in a large proportion of cases, it has an independent origin. It runs within the hepatogastric ligament along the small curvature of the stomach; it anastomoses with the right gastric artery, a branch of the hepatic artery proper.

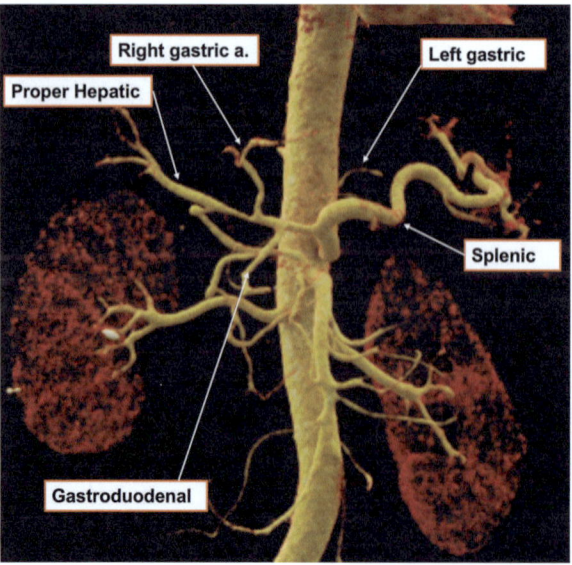

Fig. 1.8 Celiac trunk and main branches. VR reconstruction

1 Anatomy and Standardized Terminology

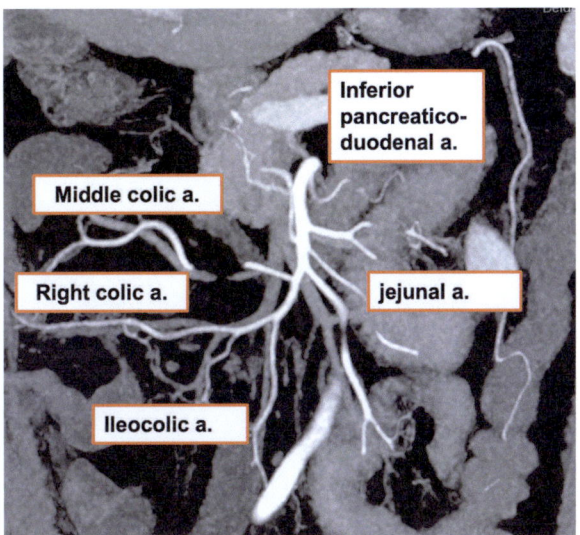

Fig. 1.9 AMS and its main branches

Common gastrohepatic or hepatic artery: after a short course it divides into: gastroduodenal artery, which in turn gives rise to the right gastroepiploic artery and the superior pancreatic-duodenal artery (which anastomoses with the inferior pancreatic-duodenal artery, a branch of the superior mesenteric artery); hepatic artery proper, from which the cystic artery originates and from which the right gastric artery may originate.

Superior mesenteric artery (AMS): originates at the level of L2–L3. It gives rise, as the first branch, to the inferior pancreatic-duodenal artery which anastomoses with the superior pancreatic-duodenal artery, a branch of the gastroduodenal artery. Further, downstream it gives rise to jejunal and ileal branches on the left side, ileocolic artery, right colic artery and middle colic artery on the right side (Fig. 1.9).

Inferior mesenteric artery (AMI): originates at the level of L3–L4. It gives rise to the left colic artery, sigmoid arteries (two to four), and the superior rectal artery.

Median sacral artery: it descends in the midline, anterior to the fourth and fifth lumbar vertebrae, sacrum, and coccyx, and ends in the coccygeal body.

Side Branches

Middle adrenal artery: it is one of the three adrenal arteries that irrigate the adrenal gland. It originates from the aorta on each side between the inferior phrenic artery and the renal artery. It courses laterally along the diaphragmatic dome.

Inferior phrenic artery: it originates from the abdominal aorta/celiac trunk and irrigates the diaphragm. It is often responsible for the extrahepatic vascularization of a hepatocellular carcinoma. It heads anteriorly and superiorly at the level of the diaphragmatic hiatus near the medial border of the adrenal gland, along the lower surface of the diaphragm (Fig. 1.10).

Renal arteries: originate at L1–L2 level, immediately downstream of the emergence of the AMS. Accessory renal arteries are often present (Fig. 1.11).

Fig. 1.10 Phrenic arteries. Axial MIP reconstruction

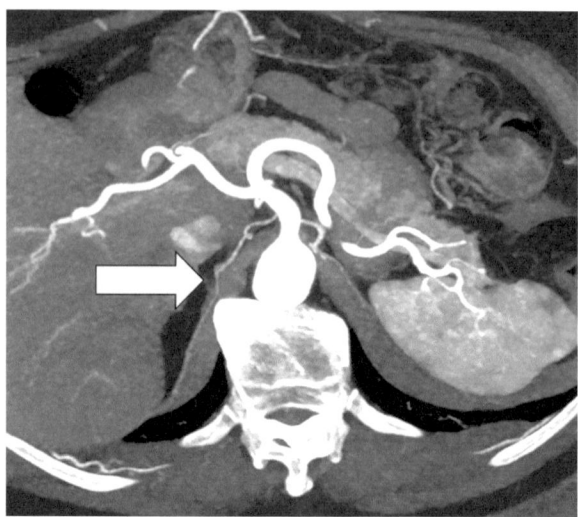

Fig. 1.11 Renal arteries. Axial MIP reconstruction

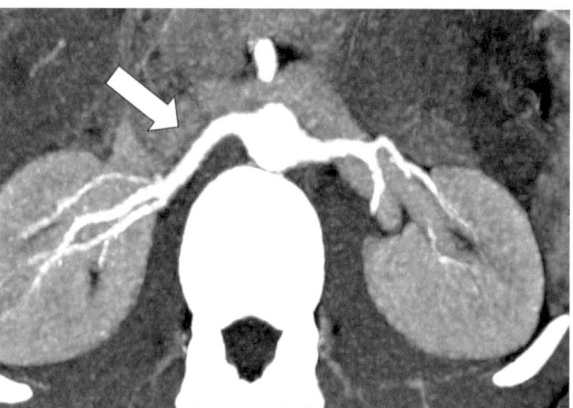

Gonadal arteries: originate at the level of L2–L3. They constitute the primary vascular supply of the ovaries and testes. They run in the retroperitoneal space and in the distal subperitoneal tract.

Lumbar arteries: they run posterolaterally along the vertebral bodies, to the right behind the inferior vena cava. After passing through the quadratus lumborum muscle, they run between the transverse muscle of the abdomen and the internal oblique muscles (Fig. 1.12).

Adamkiewicz's artery: also known as the great anterior radiculomidullary artery or arteria radicularis anterior magna, it is the name given to the dominant thoracolumbar segmental artery that irrigates the spinal cord. It arises from the radiculomidullary branch of the posterior branch of the intercostal or lumbar artery, which originates from the thoracic or abdominal aorta, respectively. It has a diameter of approximately 0.8–1.3 mm. It runs along the anterior surface of the spinal cord and

1 Anatomy and Standardized Terminology

Fig. 1.12 Lumbar arteries. Axial MIP reconstruction

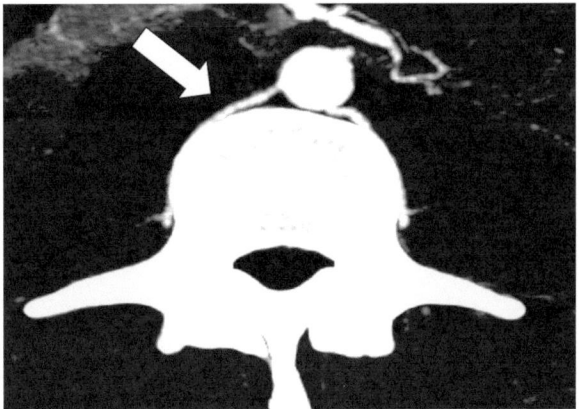

anastomoses with the anterior spinal artery through a characteristic "hairpin". The origin of the Adamkiewicz artery is quite variable and may extend from the mid-thoracic to the lumbar level. The vascular territory of the distal anterior spinal cord is at risk of ischemia or infarction if there is damage to the Adamkiewicz artery from acute aortic pathology or on an iatrogenic basis.

References

1. Magagna P, Caro R, Macchi V. Anatomia topografica dell'aorta toracica, dell'arteria ascellare e dell'arteria femorale Aorta ascendente. In: Magagna P (a cura di). Patologia dell'aorta toracica: trattamento chirurgico ed endovascolare. Piccin 2012.
2. Evangelista A, Flachskampf FA, Erbel R, et al. European Association of Echocardiography. Echocardiography in aortic diseases: EAE recommendations for clinical practice. Eur J Echocardiogr. 2010;11(8):645–58. Erratum in: Eur J Echocardiogr 2011; 12(8):642.
3. McComb BL, Munden RF, Duan F. Normative reference values of thoracic aortic diameter in American College of Radiology Imaging Network (ACRIN 6654) arm of National Lung Screening Trial. Clin Imaging. 2016;40:936–43.
4. Clemente CD. Clemente's anatomy: a regional atlas of the human body. 3rd ed. Baltimore: Urban & Schwarzenberg; 1987.
5. Standring S. Gray's anatomy: the anatomical basis of clinical practice. 39th ed. Amsterdam: Elsevier; 2004.
6. Covey AM, Brody LA, Maluccio MA, et al. Variant hepatic arterial anatomy revisited: digital subtraction angiography performed in 600 patients. Radiology. 2002;224(2):542–7.
7. Winston CB, Lee NA, Jarnagin WR, et al. CT angiography for delineation of celiac and superior mesenteric artery variants in patients undergoing hepatobiliary and pancreatic surgery. AJR Am J Roentgenol. 2007;189(1):W13–9.

Aortic Study Technique: Angio-TC: Minimum Criteria and State of the Art

2

Federica Giulio, Nicola Panvini, and Marco Rengo

CT Technical Requirements

CT studies of the thoraco-abdominal aorta can be performed with machines of any generation, although the use of modern equipment allows a reduction in both acquisition times and radiation dose to which the patient is exposed. A fundamental requirement for a high-quality study is the correct synchronization between image acquisition and the passage of the bolus of contrast medium (mdc) inside the aorta. From a technical point of view, the factor that most influences the quality of the examination is the acquisition speed. The latter is determined by three parameters: the rotation time of the X-ray tube inside the gantry, the pitch, and the size of the detector.

Rotation Time

In the spiral acquisitions, used for CT angiographic studies, the images are reconstructed with an algorithm that foresees the acquisition of data in half the rotation time of the X-ray tube-detector system; consequently, at each complete rotation of the detector, two images per detector element are reconstructed. To calculate the temporal resolution, it will be sufficient to divide the detector rotation time by two: for example, for a rotation time of 330 ms, the temporal resolution is 165 ms (Table 2.1). A high temporal resolution allows images to be acquired more quickly, limiting motion artifacts, which is particularly important in noncollaborating

---

F. Giulio · N. Panvini · M. Rengo (✉)
Department of Radiological, Oncological and Pathological Sciences, I.C.O.T. Hospital, "Sapienza" University of Rome, Latina, LT, Italy
e-mail: marco.rengo@uniroma1.it

© The Author(s), under exclusive license to Springer Nature Switzerland AG 2024
I. Carbone et al. (eds.), *Imaging of the Aorta*,
https://doi.org/10.1007/978-3-031-52527-8_2

Table 2.1 CT acquisition parameters according to the scanner

Row	Anatomical coverage (cm)	Rotation time (ms)	Temporal resolution (ms)
64	4	350	175
128	4	300	150
256	8	270	135
320	16	350	175
64-DSCT	2.4	330	83
128-DSCT	4	280	75

patients. Currently, time resolutions of less than 160 milliseconds (ms) are the standard for high-quality examinations.

Pitch

Pitch is defined as the ratio of table displacement to gantry rotation, divided by the beam width (collimation). High pitches allow to reduce the acquisition time with a consequent decrease in both the radiation dose delivered and the amount of MDC needed. At the same time, however, the increase in pitch leads to an increase in noise, and a consequent degradation of the image quality. The use of high pitches (higher than 1.3) must therefore be compensated by the use of reconstruction algorithms capable of reducing noise (iterative reconstructions).

Detector Dimensions

The detector is composed of a variable number of elements each of which has a sub-millimeter size (varying between 0.5 mm and 0.625 mm). A minimum of 16 detectors is required for the acquisition of an angio-CT examination. The size of the detector influences the acquisition time: a larger size corresponds to a larger portion of the body volume studied in a single rotation.

The dimensions of the detector are calculated by multiplying the number of elements by the thickness of each single element (e.g., 64 elements of 0.625 mm: detector dimensions = 4 cm) (Table 2.1).

The dual-source devices, being equipped with two detectors, as well as two X-ray tubes, allow to increase the anatomical coverage by doubling the anatomical volume acquired in a single rotation.

Acquisition Techniques

In the study of the thoracic aorta, motion artifacts due to cardiac pulsatility can be a problem because, especially at the level of the ascending aorta, they mimic pathologies that are not really present (e.g., intimal flap or dissection). Furthermore, cardiac movement determines a significant variability in the correct measurement of aortic

Table 2.2 Phases of cardiac cycle and imaging reconstructions

Heart rate	R-R interval	Window of acquisition (% of R-R)
50 bpm	1200 ms	60%–76% (diastole)
60 bpm	1000 ms	60%–76% (diastole)
70 bpm	857 ms	30%–77%
80 bpm	750 ms	31%–47% (systole)
90 bpm	666 ms	31%–47% (systole)

diameters, which can be as much as 18%. Therefore, for the study of the ascending aorta, it is recommended to use cardiosynchronized acquisitions with prospective or retrospective gating, which allow to minimize cardiac motion artifacts. Prospective gating involves the acquisition of images during a certain phase of the cardiac cycle, predetermined on the basis of the patient's heart rate obtained by recording the ECG tracing before acquisition (Table 2.2).

This technique involves the execution of axial scans performed with a "step and shoot" method after one or more periodic delays corresponding to the phase of the cycle chosen. The acquisition of images through prospective gating allows a drastic reduction of the radiation dose delivered to the patient, since the time of radiation emission is reduced. Moreover, this type of acquisitions allows to avoid artifacts from incorrect interpolation typical of spiral algorithms. However, this technique is severely influenced by heart rate variations and the heart rate itself, because it is based on the calculation of the chosen phase of the R-R interval during one beat and the acquisition of images at the next beat. Consequently, a prerequisite for obtaining images of suitable quality is the maintenance of a stable heart rate during the entire scan. Depending on the type of CT equipment used, there is also a heart rate limit beyond which it is not recommended to use this technique. For machines with a temporal resolution higher than ms165 this limit is 50–60 bpm. Equipment with a lower temporal resolution allows the acquisition of excellent quality images even in patients with higher heart rates if stable (with minimum variability). Retrospective gating, on the other hand, involves the continuous acquisition of images with a spiral technique throughout the cardiac cycle. Data are then retrospectively reconstructed by combining those that have the same relationship to the electrocardiographic trace, but are derived from different heartbeats allowing reconstruction of motionless images. Acquisition with retrospective gating exposes the patient to a higher radiation dose than prospective gating because of the longer emission time of the radiation itself, but has the advantage of being less sensitive to heart rate variations. Also for this type of acquisition there is a limit related to the heart rate variable according to the temporal resolution. Machines with high temporal resolution (>165 ms) allow images to be acquired in patients with heart rates no higher than 65 bpm, while lower time resolutions allow the examination to be performed even at high heart rates (>80 bpm) [1].

With the advent of dual-source equipment, a third technique has been developed, high-pitch spiral prospective gating (flash), which involves acquisition of the entire cardiac volume in a single R-R interval, allowing a drastic reduction in the radiation dose delivered to the patient. This type of acquisition is relatively insensitive to heart rate variations, but has a maximum limit of bpm60 beyond which its use is not recommended [2].

Radiation Dose Reduction Techniques

The acquisition parameter that most influences the radiation dose delivered to the patient is the kilovoltage (kV). The relationship between kV and radiation dose delivered to the patient is exponential. Consequently, a reduction in kV results in a large reduction in radiation dose. Although this leads to an increase in image noise, in angiographic studies this is a negligible problem since parenchyma evaluation is not required. Furthermore, a decrease in kV corresponds to an increase in mdc attenuation, which for angiographic studies is an advantage.

Another parameter that influences the radiation dose delivered to the patient is the milliamperage (mAs), which is the product of exposure time and the current delivered by the X-ray tube. The correlation between radiation dose and mAs is linear: a reduction in mAs therefore results in a less important decrease in radiation dose than that obtained with a reduction in kV. A reduction in mAs also leads to an increase in image noise; the reduction is then modulated along the z-axis of the patient considering changes in attenuation based on patient thickness. In retrospective acquisitions, mAs are also modulated during the cardiac cycle, in relation to the phase of the cardiac cycle predetermined for image reconstruction. For low heart rates, in which telediastole allows for high-quality image reconstruction, mAs are delivered at their maximum in this phase and reduced in the others, which are not suitable for image reconstruction [3, 4].

Contrast Medium Injection Protocols

The protocol of mdc delivery should be optimized according to the scanning protocol used. First, the iodine delivery rate (IDR) suitable to achieve an intravascular attenuation greater than 300 Hounsfield units (HU) must be identified. The choice of IDR is influenced by the kV value used for acquisition. A reduction in kV results in an increase in the attenuation of photons by iodine, leading to an increase in intravascular attenuation [5, 6]. For 120 kV acquisitions, an IDR of 2 g of iodine per second (gI/s) is recommended, with 100 kV of 1.6 gI/s and with 80 kV of 1.2 gI/s. The formula for calculating the IDR is as follows:

$$IDR = ([I]/1000) \times FR$$

where [I] is the iodine concentration per mL of mdc (expressed in mgI/mL) and FR is the injection flow (expressed in mL/s). Table 2.3 illustrates the IDR values based on mdc concentration and injection flow rate.

Once the IDR, and thus the injection flow rate, has been determined, the amount of mdc required must be determined. This is influenced by the scan time, calculated according to this formula:

$$\text{injection time} = \text{scan time} + \text{acquisition delay}$$

Table 2.3 Contrast media injection protocol

		120 kV	100 kV	80 kV
	IDR (gI/s)	2	1.6	1.2
CM concentration (mgI/mL)	270	7.4	5.9	4.4
	300	6.7	5.3	4.0
	320	6.3	5.0	3.8
	350	5.7	4.6	3.4
	370	5.4	4.3	3.2
	400	5.0	4.0	3.0
	mgI/mL	mL/s		

The acquisition delay is the time between the achievement of a predefined density value that is measured in the vascular district under examination and the beginning of the scan. Density is measured with the bolus tracking technique, which involves real-time monitoring of the passage of the bolus of mdc, or with the bolus test technique, which involves the administration of a small bolus of mdc before the main injection [7]. In both cases, the transit time of mdc from the injection site to the vascular district to be studied is determined. The commonly used threshold value (trigger value) is 100 HU. Once this value has been reached (or once the time for reaching it has been established in the case of the bolus test), the scan must begin with a delay of 8 s to avoid the acquisition of images being faster than the passage of the bolus of mdc. Knowing the acquisition time, it is possible to calculate the quantity of mdc needed with the following formula:

$$\text{volume of mdc} = \text{FR} \times (\text{scan time} + \text{acquisition delay})$$

For example, an IDR equal to 2 gI/s for an mdc with a concentration of 400 mgI/mL corresponds to a FR of 5 mL/s; if the scan lasts 6 s, the injection time will be 6 + 8 s of acquisition delay, then 14 s; multiplying (5FR) by 14 (injection time) we obtain the 70 mL dose of mdc.

After the injection of the mdc bolus, it is necessary to inject a bolus of fixed solution (approximately 50 mL) at the same flow as the mdc bolus, to compact the bolus itself and, in the case of the study of the thoracic aorta, to reduce artifacts caused by residual highly concentrated mdc in the supra-aortic venous vessels that would limit the visualization of the aortic arch and the emergence of the epiaortic vessels [8–10].

References

1. Laghi A, Rengo M. "Introduction" and "Image reconstruction". In: Cardio-CT, vol. 4. Berlin: Springer ABC; 2012.
2. Francone M, Carbone I, Danti M, et al. ECG-gated multi-detector row spiral CT in the assessment of myocardial infarction: correlation with non-invasive angiographic findings. Eur Radiol. 2006;16(1):15–24.
3. Francone M, Di Castro E, Napoli A, et al. Dose reduction and image quality assessment in 64-detector row computed tomography of the coronary arteries using an automatic exposure control system. J Comput Assist Tomogr. 2008;32(5):668–78.

4. Lambert J, MacKenzie JD, Cody D, et al. Techniques and tactics for optimizing CT dose in adults and children: state of the art and future advances. J Am Coll Radiol. 2014;11(3):262–6.
5. Caruso D, Eid M, Schoepf J, et al. Optimizing contrast media injection protocols in computed tomography angiography at different tube voltages: evaluation in a circulation phantom. J Comput Assist Tomogr. 2017;41(5):804–10.
6. Fleischmann U, Pietsch H, Korporaal JG, et al. Impact of contrast media concentration on low-kilovolt computed tomography angiography: a systematic preclinical approach. Invest Radiol. 2018;53(5):264–70.
7. Osimani M, Rengo M, Paolantonio P, et al. Sixty-four-multidetector-row computed tomography angiography with bolus tracking to time arterial-phase imaging in healthy liver: is there a correlation between quantitative and qualitative scores? J Comput Assist Tomogr. 2010;4(6):883–91.
8. Lell M, Anders K, Uder M, et al. New techniques in CT angiography. Radiographics. 2006;26(Suppl 1):S45–62.
9. Lell M, Jost G, Korporaal JG, et al. Optimizing contrast media injection protocols in state-of-the art computed tomographic angiography. Invest Radiol. 2015;50(3):161–7.
10. Rengo M, Dharampal A, Lubbers M, et al. Impact of iodine concentration and iodine delivery. Rate on contrast enhancement in coronary CT angiography: a randomized multicenter trial (CT-CON). Eur Radiol. 2019;29(11):6109–18.

MR-Angiography: Basic and Optional Sequences

3

Placido Romeo, Antonio Celona, and Maria Cristina Inserra

MR Angiographic Techniques with Intravenous Administration of Contrast Medium

Techniques involving post-contrast imaging of the aorta can be designed:

- to obtain high spatial image resolution, commonly referred to as Contrast-Enhanced Magnetic Resonance Angiography (CE-MRA);
- alternatively, to have a high temporal resolution, in which case they are defined Time-Resolved MRA (TR-MRA).

CE-MRA sequences are generally obtained by 3D Gradient technique (3D GRE), sufficiently fast to allow acquisition of an entire volume during a single apnea. They are strongly T1-weighted and are generally acquired at the conclusion of an MRI study of the aorta (Table 3.1).

Blood signal, whose T1 is strongly reduced by gadolinium, will be hyperintense regardless of the type and velocity of the flow.

The amount of gadolinium to be used is 0.1 mL/kg of body weight and is administered at a high flow rate (2–5 mL/s) [1].

P. Romeo (✉)
UOC Radiologia San Marco, AOU Policlinico "G. Rodolico", San Marco, Catania, Italy
e-mail: p.romeo@policlinico.unict.it

A. Celona
UOC Radiologia, AO Papardo, Messina, Italy
e-mail: antonio.celona@alice.it

M. C. Inserra
UOSD Radiologia CAST, AOU Policlinico "G. Rodolico", San Marco, Catania, Italy

© The Author(s), under exclusive license to Springer Nature Switzerland AG 2024
I. Carbone et al. (eds.), *Imaging of the Aorta*,
https://doi.org/10.1007/978-3-031-52527-8_3

Table 3.1 Diagnostic algorithms and main indications

Pathology	CM	Sequences	Plane	Advantages
All	No	Scout	Axial/coronal/sagittal	
	No	Cine b SSFP retro	Axial on chest and/or aortic valve	Evaluation of valvular morphology
	No	Cine b SSFP retro	Axial/para-sagittal (Candy Stick)	Evaluation of fluxes, wall and flap
Stenosis, insufficiency	No	PC through plane	Perpendicular to aortic valve and ST junction	Evaluation of fluxes for stenosis or valvular insufficiency
Aneurysm, coarctation, congenital anomalies	No	3D T1 FS gated (systole)	Volumetric, thoracic aorta	Evaluation of walls and diameters
	No	3D whole heart gated (diastole)	Volumetric, thoracic aorta	Evaluation of anatomy for congenital anomalies
Vasculitis	No	TSE T2 FS	Axial, coronal, Para-sagittal	Evaluation of edema within the wall
	Yes	3DT1 GRE in breath-hold	Volumetric, thoracic aorta	Evaluation of hypervascularization of the wall
Dissection, stenosis, coarctation, thrombosis	Yes	CE-MRA	Volumetric, thoracic aorta	Evaluation of vascular lumen
Dissection for flap evaluation	Yes	TR-MRA	Volumetric, thoracic aorta	Evaluation of dissection flaps and fluxes

To synchronize the timing of the acquisition with the CM transit, the bolus tracking technique or, alternatively, MRI fluoroscopy can be used. In the first case, the sequence starts automatically when a certain signal intensity of the blood, preset by the operator, is reached within a region of interest (ROI); in the second case, after the intravenous infusion of the CM, rapid images are acquired with 2D GRE technique of the reference anatomical region and the start of the sequence is manually activated when the CM transit is visualized. The images thus obtained can be reprocessed on a workstation using different reconstruction algorithms (MIP, MPR or Volume Rendering) (Fig. 3.1a).

TR-MRA sequences (TRICKS, TWIST, 4D-TRACK, TRAQ or Freeze Frame, depending on the vendor) offer the possibility of making very fast acquisitions, useful for demonstrating the transit of CM in the various vascular structures under study. They are 3D spoiled GRE sequences that, in order to obtain this result, acquire more often the central zone of K-space (Keyhole Imaging), related to image contrast information.

The latter information is completed with that obtained from a high resolution mask (View Sharing), acquired before the administration of the CM. This technique, which is a useful complement to CE-MRA, allows to evaluate not only the progression of the CM but also the possible presence of collateral circles, inhomogeneous flows or dissections, being extremely useful in correctly discriminating between true and false lumen of the vessel (Fig. 3.1b).

3 MR-Angiography: Basic and Optional Sequences

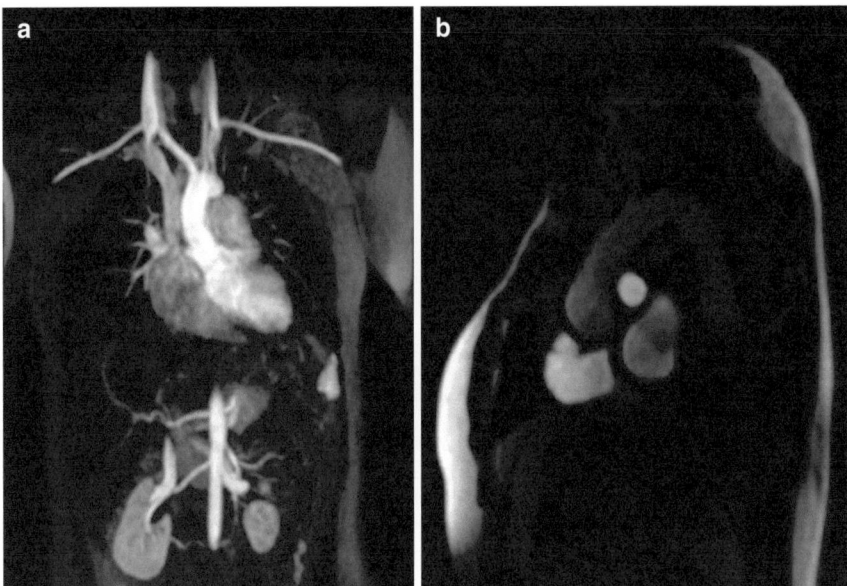

Fig. 3.1 (**a**) CE-MRA acquisition with MIP post-processing reconstruction in the coronal plane; (**b**) TR-MRA acquisition in a parasagittal plane for visualization of the aortic arch. The signal intensity of the moving blood is modified according to the transit time of the mdc in the cardiac cavities

Bright Blood MR Angiography Techniques

Steady State Free Precession (SSFP), Time Of Flight (TOF), and Phase-Contrast (PC) angiographic sequences can be considered in this group.

SSFP sequences (TrueFISP, Balanced-FFE or FIESTA, depending on the Vendors) are extremely versatile as they allow fast imaging, with apneas of 5–6 s taking advantage of very low TR and TE and parallel imaging [2] (Fig. 3.2a).

The images obtained have good spatial resolution, high contrast resolution, high SNR even on large Field of View (FOV). The constant hypersignal of the blood allows to evaluate the valvular and wall alterations and to exclude the possible presence of dissections. These sequences can generate static or cine images. They allow synchronization with ECG and/or respiratory gating, but can be also effected by a non ECG-gated real-time free-breathing technique.

Static 3D free-breathing volumetric packages (3D Whole Heart Imaging) can be acquired, with cardiac and respiratory gating for good anatomical assessment of the district under examination [3] (Fig. 3.2b). However, SSFPs have a high susceptibility to magnetic field alterations such as those caused by the presence of metal prostheses or stents. The cines are sometimes found to be extremely sensitive to turbulent flows that infirms the diagnostic image quality (Fig. 3.2c).

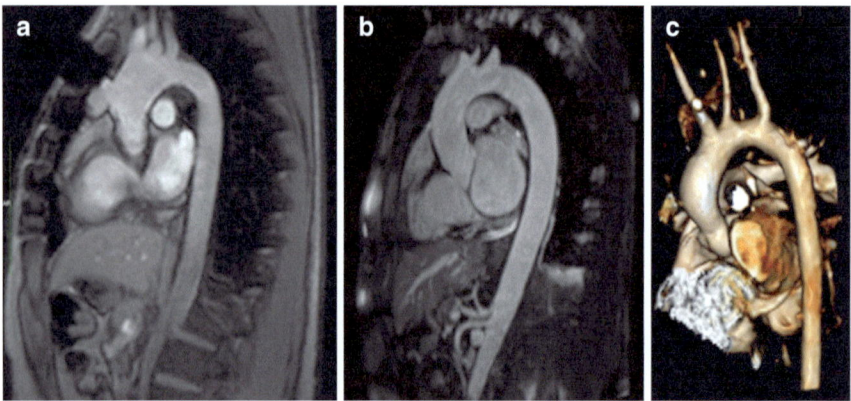

Fig. 3.2 (**a**) SSFP "Candy Stick" acquisition of the ascending aorta in a patient with pseudo-aneurysm at the level of the insertion of a venous graft on the anterior wall of ascending aorta; (**b**) MIP reconstruction from 3D Whole Heart sequence; (**c**) Volume Rendering

TOF sequences are currently seldom used in the study of the aorta because of their susceptibility to respiratory and cardiac movements. Moreover limitations due to saturation, large FOVs used, aortic course and curvatures generate low quality images.

PC sequences [4] provide information on speed and volume of blood flow inside the vessel. They play a major role in cases where discrepancy emerges between the flows of the various sections of the cardiovascular system as in the presence of left-right shunt, in patients with congenital heart disease, or in evaluation of collateral circles in cases of aortic coarctation. They take advantage of the application of a bipolar gradient along the phase axis. Stationary tissues have a zeroing of the phase shift at the finish of gradient application, while blood signal due to its flow through imaged section, will have a net deflection that depends on its speed.

Flows of equal velocity, with opposite directions, will have equal magnitude of deflection of the spins but opposite phase. We can thus assess flow velocity within a vascular section and determine the flow rate of the vessel. The amplitude, duration, and spacing between gradients allow the sequence to be sensible at different flow speeds, which should be indicated in the Velocity Encoding parameter (VENC), selectable by the operator. The use of VENC values lower than those of the presumed blood velocity inside investigated vessel results in the appearance of aliasing artifacts, as the velocity curve above the established VENC is considered to be as having opposite flow direction (Fig. 3.3). In contrast, too high values of selected VENC infit the accuracy of the measured flow speed.

Magnitude and phase images are obtained, in apnea or free breath, with or without cardiac gating, demonstrating the flow trend during the entire study interval (such as during an R-R interval on the ECG).

PCs can be 2D, 3D, or 4D sequences. With regard to the study of the aorta 2D and 4D ones are used. The latter (4D-Flow), recently introduced, allow acquisition of a free-breathing volumetric package, which can be reprocessed on a workstation.

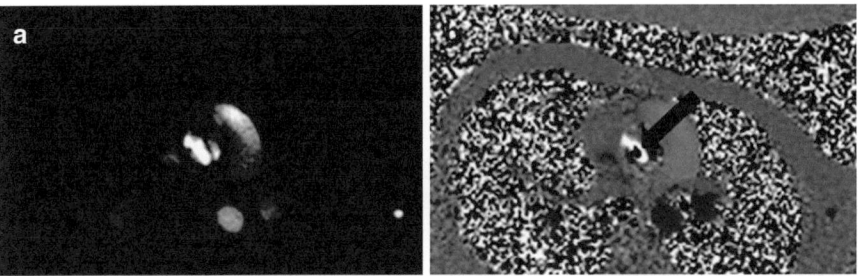

Fig. 3.3 PC through plane acquisition on the aortic valve plane. (**a**) Magnitude image; (**b**) phase image, where aliasing related to an incorrect VENC value (arrow) can be appreciated

Information on the flows can be obtained by choosing the section to be investigated ex-post and obtain useful information on the direction and the types of flows, as well as on the stress to which the vascular walls are subjected, which may be predictive of their remodeling [5].

Black Blood MR Angiographic Techniques

Under this name are included RM techniques characterized by moving blood signal saturation so resulting "black." These are conventional or echo-train spin echo sequences (TSE, FSE, depending on the vendor); they can be acquired in apnea of free-breathing, with or without cardiac gating. Echo-train techniques are preferred as they allow the acquisition of the package during a single apnea. In case of particularly compromised patient they can be substituted by single-shot acquisitions (HASTE, SS-FSE, SSH-TSE, FASE or single-shot fast SE) which have good quality also in free breath.

They have the ability to enhance the contrast between the moving blood and the vessel wall and are useful in highlighting intramural changes such as hematoma, flap and thrombotic apposition [1]. The 90° gradient is not applied to moving blood, nor is the subsequent "refocusing" gradient applied as it transits through the thickness of the slice under investigation (washout effect), resulting in signal abatement. Slow flows or vascular occlusions can result in signal inside the vessel walls.

Generally, black blood techniques are used to integrate the information obtained with other white blood angiographic techniques, with or without the use of CM. In these sequences the turbulent flows, which cause an overestimation of stenosis in bright blood, contribute to the improvement of the difference of signal between lumen and vascular wall. In addition, with the suppression of the blood signal no pulsation artifacts (ghosting) are appreciated; the vessel walls are therefore perfectly contrasted with respect to the lumen.

Acquisitions can be T1- or T2-weighted and obtained 2D or 3D techniques. T2-weighted images with fat suppression can highlight wall edema and aid in the diagnosis of vasculitis [6]. Useful for the assessment of aortic diameters appear to be 3D T1 acquisitions with cardiac and respiratory gating [7] (Fig. 3.4).

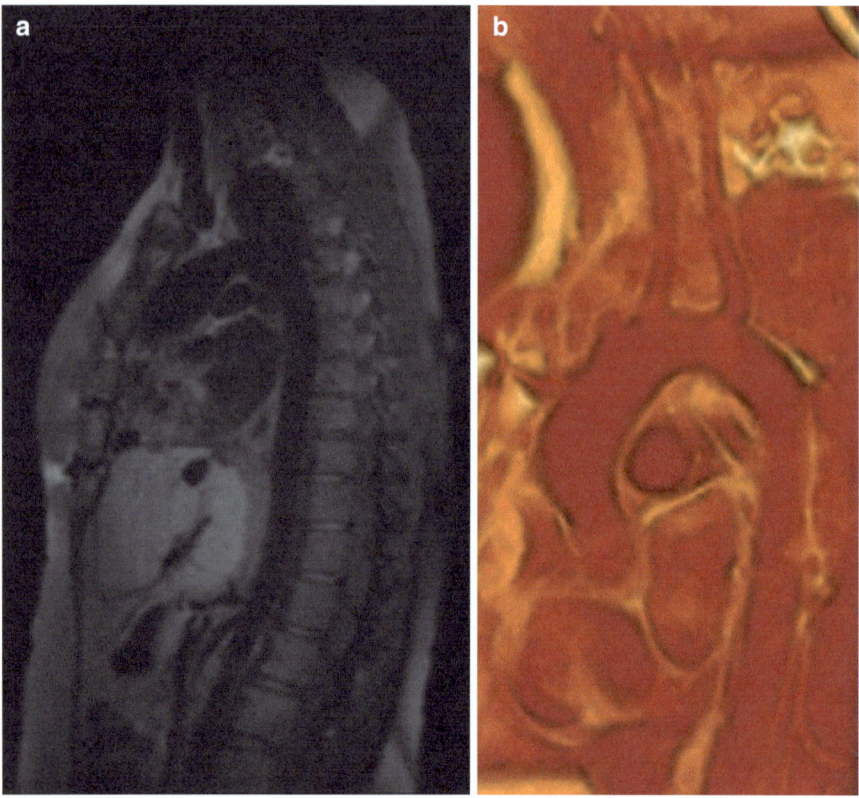

Fig. 3.4 3D T1 black blood acquisition. (**a**) Parasagittal MPR reconstruction; (**b**) Volume Rendering

To convert a set of 3D black blood images into an angiographic acquisition, one must use minimum-intensity projection (MinIP) reconstruction algorithms on the post-processing workstation.

Evaluation of Chest Structures

If it is necessary to study the perivascular thoracic structures, the examination can be integrated with single-shot T2 acquisitions and with pre-contrast 3D GRE sequences, performed in axial or coronal planes with a minimum increase in acquisition time. If necessary, after CE-MRA an additional 3D GRE post-contrast package can be acquired to visualize the lungs and other anatomical structures of the chest.

References

1. Herédia V, Ramalho M, Duarte S, et al. Magnetic resonance imaging of the thoracic aorta: a review of technical and clinical aspects, including its use in the evaluation of aneurysms and acute vascular conditions. London: IntechOpen; 2011. https://doi.org/10.5772/21835.
2. Sakamoto I, Sueyoshi E, Uetani M. MR imaging of the aorta. Radiol Clin North Am. 2007;45(3):485–97, viii.
3. Krishnam MS, Tomasian A, Deshpande V, et al. Noncontrast 3D steady-state free-precession. Magnetic resonance angiography of the whole chest using nonselective radiofrequency excitation over a large field of view: comparison with single-phase 3D contrast-enhanced magnetic resonance angiography. Invest Radiol. 2008;43(6):411–20.
4. Hom JJ, Ordovas K, Reddy GP. Velocity-encoded cine MR imaging in aortic coarctation: functional assessment of hemodynamic events. Radiographics. 2008;28(2):407–16.
5. Bhave NM, Nienaber CA, Clough RE, Eagle KA. Multimodality imaging of thoracic aortic diseases in adults. JACC Cardiovasc Imaging. 2018;11(6):902–19.
6. Quinn KA, Ahlman MA, Malayeri AA, et al. Comparison of magnetic resonance angiography and 18F-fluorodeoxyglucose positron emission tomography in large-vessel vasculitis. Ann Rheum Dis. 2018;77(8):1165–71.
7. Eikendal ALM, Blomberg BA, Haaring C, et al. 3D black blood VISTA vessel wall cardiovascular magnetic resonance of the thoracic aorta wall in young, healthy adults: reproducibility and implications for efficacy trial sample sizes: a cross-sectional study. J Cardiovasc Magn Reson. 2016;18:20.

Transthoracic and Transesophageal Echocardiography

4

Elena Cavarretta

Transthoracic Echocardiography

It is the most widely used method for assessing the size, thickness, and systolic-diastolic function of the ventricles, the size and volume of the atria, the morphology and function of the four heart valves, the size of the great vessels, and the status of the pericardium. This examination has several clinical indications: in the presence of symptoms or abnormalities found on the ECG or other exams as well as for screening or follow-up of cardiovascular patients [1].

It allows an accurate assessment of different segments of the ascending aorta, such as the aortic bulb with the sinuses of Valsalva and the aortic valve cusps, the sino-tubular junction, the proximal ascending aorta and in most cases also the distal aortic arch and a small portion of the proximal descending aorta.

The distal ascending aorta and proximal aortic arch cannot be visualized with this method because the presence of the right main bronchus resulting in an ultrasound-blind zone.

The long axis parasternal window (Fig. 4.1) is the first projection from which an echocardiographic examination begins and allows visualization of the aortic bulb and proximal ascending aorta in longitudinal section. The left ventricular outflow tract with the aortic annulus is also appreciated, as well as two of the aortic cusps: the right coronary and non-coronary. It is by far the most useful projection for measuring the diastolic and systolic diameter of the aortic bulb at the level of the sinuses of Valsalva, the sino-tubular junction, and the proximal ascending tubular aorta. In

---

E. Cavarretta (✉)
Department of Medical-Surgical Sciences and Biotechnologies, Sapienza University of Rome, Latina, Italy
e-mail: elena.cavarretta@uniroma1.it

© The Author(s), under exclusive license to Springer Nature Switzerland AG 2024
I. Carbone et al. (eds.), *Imaging of the Aorta*,
https://doi.org/10.1007/978-3-031-52527-8_4

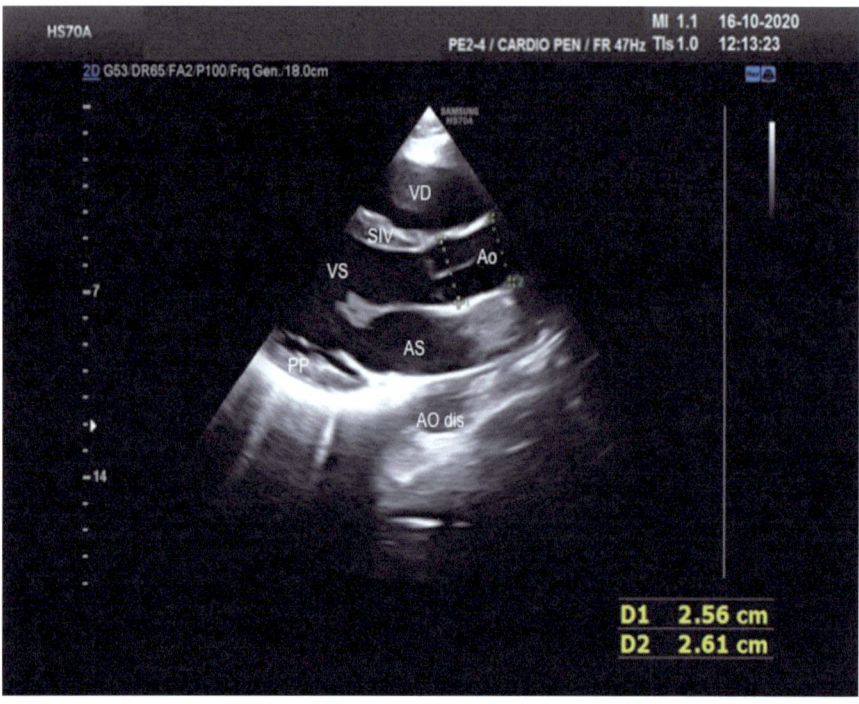

Fig. 4.1 Transthoracic echocardiography, parasternal projection long axis. The following structures can be appreciated: the aortic bulb with the sinuses of Valsalva and the aortic valve, the sinotubular junction and the ascending tubular aorta (asc TA), the left ventricle (LV), whose cavity is delimited by the posterior wall and the interventricular septum (IVS), which separates it from the right ventricle (RV). The left atrium (LA) and both mitral valve leaflets are appreciable, and below the descending thoracic aorta (des TA) is seen in cross-section

the parasternal long axis projection in cine mode, the morphology and the movement of the aortic cusps can be appreciated. In aortic bicuspidy, the cusps are typically prolapsed toward the left ventricle, or they can be sclero-calcific, with a reduced opening movement in aortic stenosis. In this projection, the presence of aortic valve regurgitation or the possible acceleration of the transvalvular flow typical of aortic valve stenosis is evaluated with the use of the color Doppler modality. In the parasternal short-axis view, there is perfect visualization of the aortic valve in cross-section and of the three aortic valve cusps (right coronary, left coronary, and non-coronary) as well as the origin of the two coronary arteries from their respective sinuses of Valsalva.

Due to the lack of alignment of the ultrasound beam, it is not possible to evaluate the kinetics of the transvalvular aortic flow from the parasternal long axis view, for

4 Transthoracic and Transesophageal Echocardiography

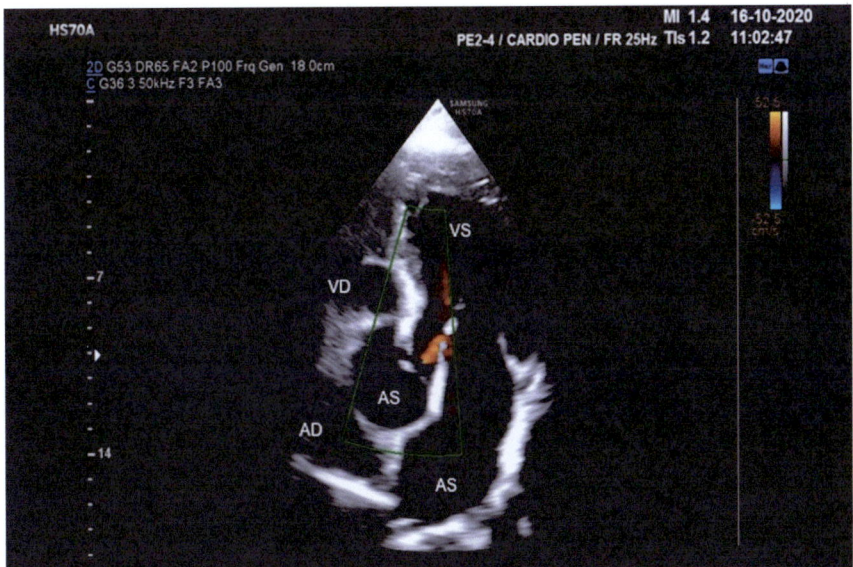

Fig. 4.2 Transthoracic echocardiography, apical chamber 5 projections. The aortic bulb (AB) is visualized; in color Doppler mode, a mild aortic valve insufficiency is appreciated. *RA* right atrium, *LA* left atrium, *RV* right ventricle, *LV* left ventricle

which it is necessary to use the apical "5-chamber" window (Fig. 4.2). This allows visualization of the cardiac chambers (the 2 atria and 2 ventricles), the aortic bulb, and the ascending aorta; it has a good alignment with the ultrasound beam and, thanks to Doppler, allows assessment of the transvalvular velocity and any flow of aortic regurgitation.

In the subcostal window, a 4- or 5-chamber projection is also appreciated, but lacking the alignment necessary to assess transvalvular flows.

The suprasternal projection is used to visualize the aortic arch and measure the velocity at the level of the isthmus, always in supine decubitus (Fig. 4.3).

Cost-effectiveness, non-invasiveness, and absence of ionizing radiation make transthoracic echocardiography particularly useful in the screening and serial evaluation of aortic pathologies such as aortic ectasia and aortic coarctation. It is the first-choice method in the evaluation of congenital heart disease, starting from intrauterine screening, since the acoustic window in children is optimal and the cooperation from the pediatric patient can be modulated. In emergency/urgent situations, such as acute aortic syndromes, transthoracic echocardiography can be diagnostic, although it often remains necessary to use another imaging modality, primarily CT angiography, for a more panoramic assessment.

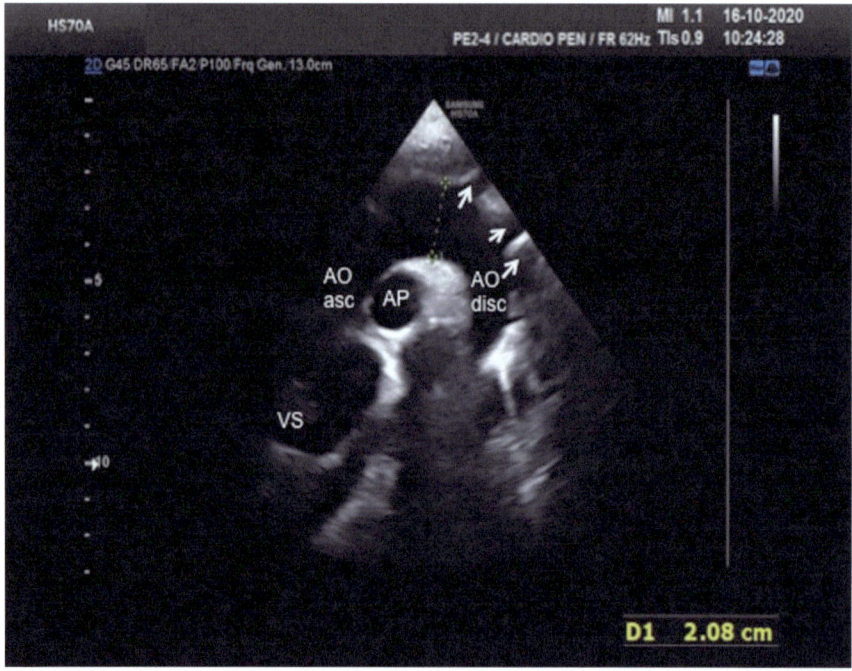

Fig. 4.3 Transthoracic echocardiography, suprasternal projection. The aortic arch is visualized in its entirety, including the origin of the supra-aortic trunks (arrows). In transverse section the Right branch of the pulmonary artery (PA). *Asc TA* ascending thoracic aorta, *des TA* descending thoracic aorta, *LV* left ventricle

Transesophageal Echocardiography

If transthoracic echocardiography offers a limited assessment of the thoracic aorta, transesophageal echocardiography (TEE) provides a complete visualization of the aorta from the aortic valve to the distal descending thoracic aorta.

Transesophageal examination is considered a semi-invasive examination because the echo-graphy probe is introduced into the esophagus. It is a very useful approach in intubated and intensive care patients, since, due to mechanical ventilation, the transthoracic acoustic window is often suboptimal. In cooperating patients, oral sedation with lidocaine spray or conscious sedation is useful for better tolerance of the exam and thus better success [1].

TEE is particularly useful in several conditions that cannot be completely assessed by TTE, including (1) the presence of cardioembolic sources (presence of intracavitary thrombus or masses); (2) the evaluation of the interatrial septum, in particular at the level of the foramen ovale; (3) the characterization of heart valves morphology and function (floppy mitral valve, bicuspid aortic valve, etc.); (4) the perioperative evaluation during cardiac surgery or percutaneous interventions;

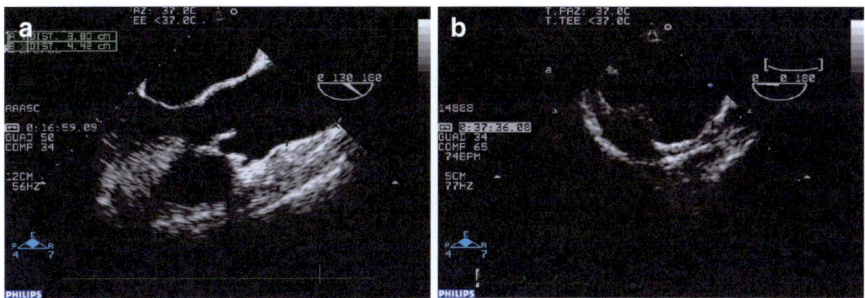

Fig. 4.4 (**a**) Mid-esophageal projection at 130°. (**b**) Mid-esophageal projection at 0°; descending thoracic aorta in cross-section with uncomplicated atheroma

(5) infective endocarditis; (6) pathologies of the ascending thoracic aorta (aneurysm, atheromasia, acute aortic syndromes) and (7) in all conditions of hemodynamic instability in the intensive care unit/operating room [2].

The transesophageal probe has a very limited mobility inside the esophagus; however, through the mid-esophageal and transgastric projections and thanks to the rotation between 0° and 180° it is possible to visualize all the structures of interest: the aortic bulb in longitudinal section and the left ventricle (Fig. 4.4a) or the aortic bulb at the level of the sinuses of Valsalva in transverse section.

In order to assess the transvalvular aortic flows with Doppler, it is necessary to use the deep transgastric projection because an excellent alignment with the bulb and ascending aorta is obtained.

Rotating the transesophageal probe by 90° provides visualization of the descending thoracic aorta, either in cross-section at 0° or in longitudinal section at 90°; when the probe is withdrawn, the entire length of the descending aorta until the aortic arch is visualized, which usually concludes the transesophageal examination. This projection is particularly useful in assessing the morphology and localization of aortic atheromasia (Fig. 4.4b) [2].

References

1. Armstrong WF, Ryan T. Feigenbaum's Echocardiography. Philadelphia, PA: Lippincott Williams & Wilkins; 2018.
2. Evangelista A, Maldonado G, Gruosso D, et al. The current role of echocardiography in acute aortic syndrome. Echo Res Pract. 2019;6(2):R53–63.

Ultrasound of the Abdominal Aorta

5

Simone Vicini, Paola Lucchesi, Marco Maria Maceroni, and Elena Orlando

Examination Technique

Given its anatomical position in the retroperitoneum, anterior to the spine and next to the inferior vena cava, adequate visualization of the abdominal aorta requires a high penetration capacity of the ultrasound beam. For this purpose, probes with low-frequency (3–5 MHz) convex geometry transducers (convex probe) are used; sometimes, in obese patients, it may be useful to extend the frequency range of transducers to 1 MHz for an adequate evaluation of the abdominal aorta [1].

The examination is performed with the patient supine, placing the probe in the epigastric region on the midline or left paramedian; the aorta is studied by longitudinal, axial or oblique scans, from the diaphragmatic hiatus to the aortic bifurcation. The morphological evaluation of the vessel is performed using the B-Mode (Brightness Mode, with modulation of the gray scale in real time): if the measure the caliber in correspondence of the major diameter (orthogonal) along the anteroposterior and transverse planes and it is possible to demonstrate any parietal alterations with a calcium component (plaques or thrombi) (Fig. 5.1).

The color Doppler module also allows a functional evaluation, because it represents the blood flow within the arterial lumen in the form of a chromatic vascular map and velocitogram, thus identifying any changes in the same (turbulence or demodulation of the flow).

Analysis of the spectrum, with the aid of the acoustic signal, allows a qualitative and quantitative assessment of the flow. The normal velocitogram of the abdominal aorta is characterized by a rapid rise in velocity finally to the systolic peak, followed by a very rapid negative phase due to parietal elasticity, followed by an anterograde diastolic flow (Fig. 5.2).

S. Vicini (✉) · P. Lucchesi · M. M. Maceroni · E. Orlando
Department of Radiological, Oncological and Pathological Sciences, I.C.O.T. Hospital, "Sapienza" University of Rome, Latina, LT, Italy

© The Author(s), under exclusive license to Springer Nature Switzerland AG 2024
I. Carbone et al. (eds.), *Imaging of the Aorta*,
https://doi.org/10.1007/978-3-031-52527-8_5

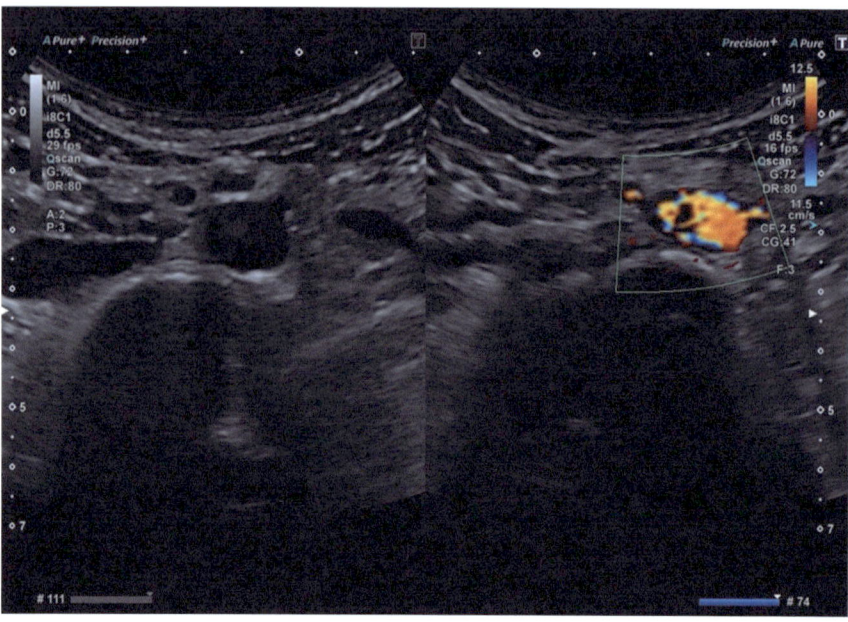

Fig. 5.1 Axial B-Mode and color Doppler scan of normal abdominal aorta

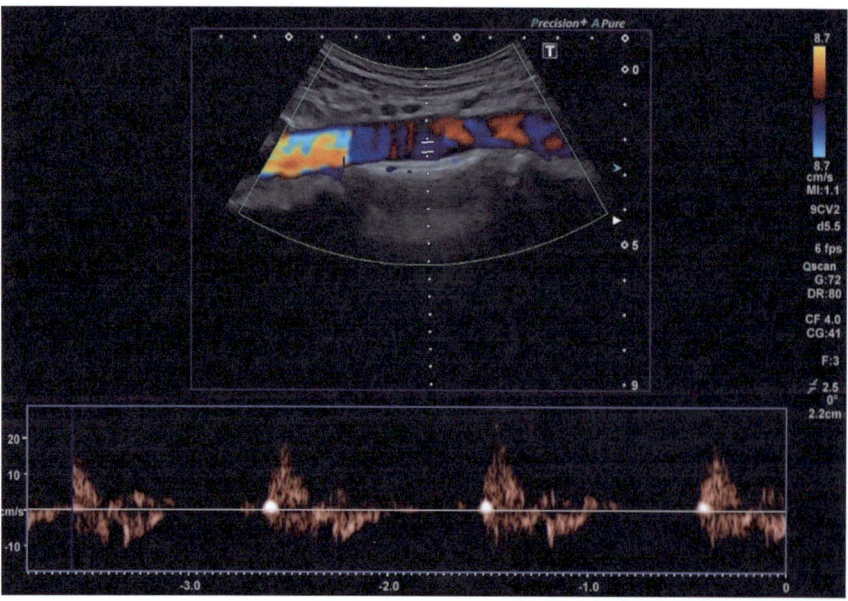

Fig. 5.2 Longitudinal scan of abdominal aorta with normal velocitogram

The limitations of the method are the general limitations of abdominal ultrasound, mainly related to obesity, intestinal meteorism, and poor patient collaboration.

Echographic Semeiotics

Aneurysm of the abdominal aorta, easily identifiable by ultrasound examination, is sometimes an occasional finding during ultrasound examinations of the abdomen performed for other indications.

The diagnosis of aortic aneurysm is made when the diameter of the aorta is more than 3 cm or when the transverse diameter in one sector is twice that of the adjacent proximal tract [2].

Morphological examination in B-Mode provides much of the information of clinical interest, such as aneurysm location, size, morphology, possible involvement of other vascular structures, and presence of complications.

Color Doppler allows the identification of pathological changes in flow within the vascular lumen and the presence of parietal thrombosis.

On ultrasound examination, the aneurysm of the abdominal aorta may present as a symmetrical dilatation involving the entire circumference of the vessel (fusiform aneurysm) or, less frequently, as a focal eccentric bulge of the wall (saccular aneurysm), which is often associated with parietal alterations of an atherosclerotic nature, represented by calcifications and thrombotic apposition.

Once an aneurysm has been identified, the main clinical aspects to be evaluated are those concerning its site, in relation to the origin of the renal arteries (i.e., suprator infrarenal localization), its distal extension, with possible involvement of the iliac arteries, and the size of the aneurysm sac in the transverse and antero-posterior planes.

In the not infrequent cases of parietal thrombotic apposition in the context of an aneurysm, the evaluation of the caliber of the residual lumen is very important: this measure allows to estimate the risk of rupture of the aneurysm, which, according to Laplace's law, is higher the greater the diameter of the pervious lumen [3]. Moreover, using the color Doppler module, a correct visualization of the pervious lumen is possible, since on morphological examination the vessel caliber may be underestimated due to the anechogenic appearance of parietal thrombotic apposition or, in extreme cases, a completely obstructed lumen may be considered pervious. In these cases, demonstration of flow within a contiguous vessel gives certainty of the absence of flow in the aorta and excludes any possibility of inappropriate device adjustment (e.g., PRF too high).

Color Doppler, in addition to detecting the presence of turbulent flow within the aneurysmal sac, also allows the detection of the possible presence of flow in the context of a parietal thrombus, a typical finding of aneurysm instability that may be a prelude to more serious complications (Fig. 5.3).

The ultrasound examination can represent a valid tool also in the preliminary evaluation of possible complications of an abdominal aortic aneurysm. The fixuration represents the most serious complication of the aneurysm, which ultrasound

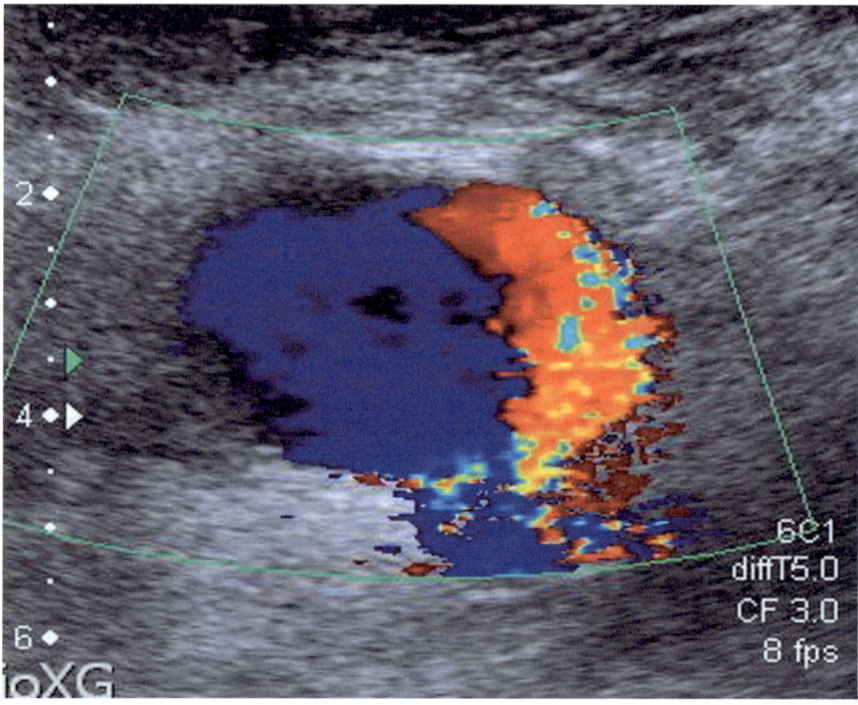

Fig. 5.3 Turbulent flow in the aneurysmal sac can be visualized on color Doppler as bidirectional flow, known as the "Yin-Yang Sign". (Case courtesy of Dr. Maciej Mazgaj, Radiopaedia.org, rID:33283)

can identify by highlighting inhomogeneities of retroperitoneal adipose tissue in the periaortic location, sometimes in the presence of gross fluid collections or hemoperitoneum. Color Doppler has not improved the sensitivity of the method in this complication, for the diagnosis of which CT has shown better diagnostic accuracy.

In cases of aortic dissection, ultrasound examination can detect flow into the true lumen and in the diastolic phase blood reflow into the false lumen. In some cases, the reentry orifice of the flow from the false lumen into the true lumen can be identified.

References

1. Schäberle W, Leyerer L, Schierling W, Pfister K. Ultrasound diagnostics of the abdominal aorta. Gefässchirurgie. 2015;20(Suppl 1):22–7.
2. Gameraddin M. Normal abdominal aorta diameter on abdominal sonography in healthy asymptomatic adults: impact of age and gender. J Radiat Res Appl Sci. 2019;12(1):186–91.
3. Chiu KW, Ling L, Tripathi V, et al. Ultrasound measurement for abdominal aortic aneurysm screening: a direct comparison of the three leading methods. Eur J Vasc Endovasc Surg. 2014;47(4):367–73.

Part II
The Aorta on the Chest X-Ray

Anatomical Landmarks: Lines and Stripes

6

Maria Dea Ippoliti, Emanuela Algeri, and Iacopo Carbone

In the evaluation of chest radiographs, it is essential to know the lines, bands, and interfaces that are demarcated between the mediastinal structures and the lungs. In the frontal chest X-ray images, approaching the radiographic study of the aorta, the following lines and interfaces have to be recognized: the *para-aortic line*: visible behind the cardiac image, lateral to the left paraspinal line, with a vertical course; it is formed by the contact between the lateral wall of the descending thoracic aorta and the lower lobe of the left lung;

- the *aorto-pulmonary* space: triangular area delimited superiorly by the aortic arch, inferiorly by the left pulmonary artery, anteriorly by the ascending aorta, posteriorly by the descending aorta, medially by the trachea, laterally by the mediastinal pleura of the left lung;
- the *left subclavian line*: visible above the aortic arch, with a slightly concave shape oriented towards the left; it is formed by the contact of the lateral wall of the left subclavian artery with the upper lobe of the left lung;
- the *right para-caval line or first cardiac arch*: it represents the right upper limit of the cardiac shadow; in young patients, it is formed by the interface between

---

M. D. Ippoliti
Department of Radiological, Oncological and Pathological Sciences, I.C.O.T. Hospital, "Sapienza" University of Rome, Latina, LT, Italy
e-mail: mariadea.ippoliti@uniroma1.it

E. Algeri (✉)
Service de Radiologie et Imagerie Cardiovasculaire, Hôpital Cardiologique, Centre Hospitalier Régional et Universitaire de Lille, Lille Cedex, France

I. Carbone
Academic Diagnostic Imaging Division, Department of Medical-Surgical Sciences and Biotechnologies, Faculty of Pharmacy and Medicine, I.C.O.T. Hospital, University of Rome "Sapienza", Latina, LT, Italy
e-mail: iacopo.carbone@uniroma1.it

© The Author(s), under exclusive license to Springer Nature Switzerland AG 2024
I. Carbone et al. (eds.), *Imaging of the Aorta*,
https://doi.org/10.1007/978-3-031-52527-8_6

the upper lobe of the right lung and the lateral edge of the superior vena cava and has a vertical course ending in the right atrium; in elder patients, it is more frequently formed by the interface between the upper lobe of the right lung and the lateral edge of the ascending thoracic aorta (often of greater caliber in the elderly) and has a slightly concave shape towards the right;
- the *inter-azygos-esophageal recess*: the interface between middle mediastinum (hypodiaphan) and the postero-medial segment of the lower lobe of the right lung (hyperdiaphan);
- the *right para-spinal line*: given by the interface between the right lung (hyperdiaphan) and the soft tissues of the posterior mediastinum (hypodiaphan);
- the *left para-spinal line*: given by the interface between the left lung (hyperdiaphan) and the soft tissues of the posterior mediastinum (hypodiaphan).

All the lines and interfaces aforementioned are described in Fig. 6.1 and Fig. 6.2.
In the lateral projection radiograph (Fig. 6.3) we recognize:

- the anterior profile of the ascending aorta;
- the superior profile of the aortic arch.

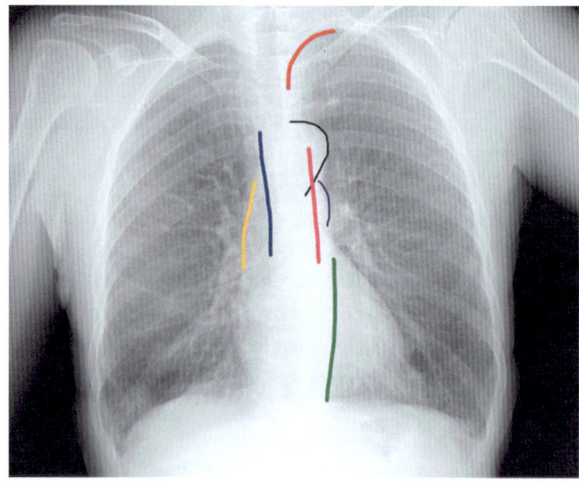

Fig. 6.1 Chest radiograph in PA projection. Green: para-aortic line; purple: aorto-pulmonary fiber; red: left subclavian line; yellow: para-caval line or right first cardiac arch; blue: right para-spinal line; pink: left para-spinal line; black: aortic arch

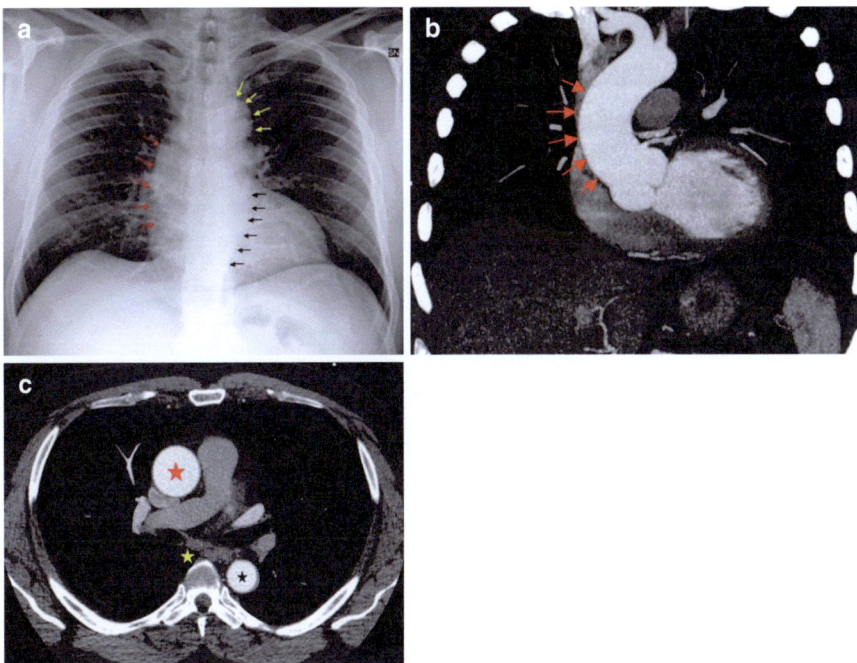

Fig. 6.2 In older patients, or in case of aortic root ectasia, the first right cardiac arch- or para-caval line (red arrows in figure **a**), shows mild convexity on the right side, consisting in the right lateral edge of the ascending aorta (red arrows in figure **b**). In figure **a**, the yellow arrows indicate the left superior cardiac arch, and the para-aortic line is indicated by the black arrows. In figure **c**, the red star indicates the ascending aorta, the black star indicates the descending aorta, and the yellow star indicates the interazygos-esophageal recess

Fig. 6.3 Chest radiograph in LL projection. Red: posterior tracheal line; purple: ascending thoracic aorta; blue: aortic arch

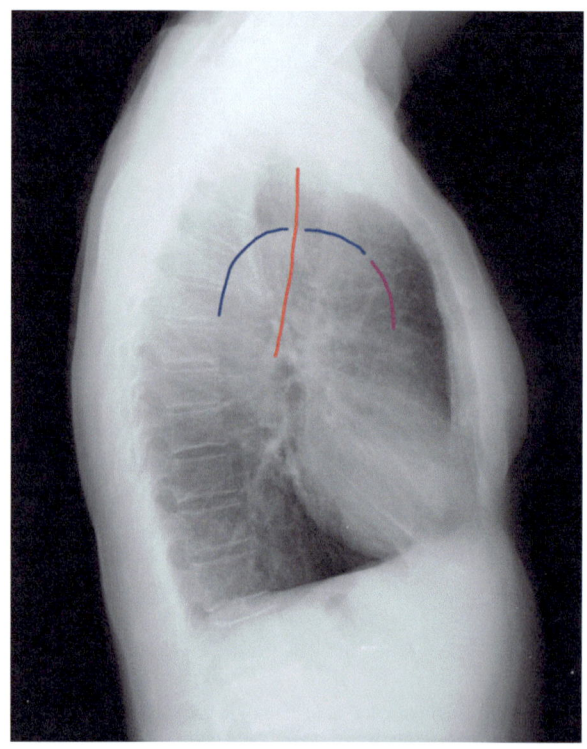

Abnormal Findings

7

Maria Dea Ippoliti, Emanuela Algeri, and Iacopo Carbone

Chest X-ray imaging is quick to perform and easily available even in small medical centres.

The suspicion of aortic pathology should be raised by a variety of radiological findings, such as shift or widening of the lines and interfaces described above, or the appearance of a silhouette sign.

The silhouette sign is defined as an opacity adjacent to mediastinal structures, with disappearance of the physiological lines and interfaces visible on chest radiograph.

Thoracic Aortic Aneurysm

In most cases it develops in the ascending thoracic aorta.

It can be seen in both the postero-anterior and latero-lateral projection as:

- widening of the second mediastinal arch (in the PA projection) or of the antero-superior profile of the mediastinum (in the LL projection);

M. D. Ippoliti (✉)
Department of Radiological, Oncological and Pathological Sciences, I.C.O.T. Hospital, "Sapienza" University of Rome, Latina, LT, Italy
e-mail: mariadea.ippoliti@uniroma1.it

E. Algeri
Service de Radiologie et Imagerie Cardiovasculaire, Hôpital Cardiologique, Centre Hospitalier Régional et Universitaire de Lille, Lille Cedex, France

I. Carbone
Academic Diagnostic Imaging Division, Department of Medical-Surgical Sciences and Biotechnologies, Faculty of Pharmacy and Medicine, I.C.O.T. Hospital, University of Rome "Sapienza", Latina, LT, Italy
e-mail: iacopo.carbone@uniroma1.it

© The Author(s), under exclusive license to Springer Nature Switzerland AG 2024
I. Carbone et al. (eds.), *Imaging of the Aorta*,
https://doi.org/10.1007/978-3-031-52527-8_7

- the aorto-pulmonary space may show a convex margin; this finding becomes more prominent when observed as a new finding in comparison with previous frontal chest X-ray images;
- abnormal thickening of the posterior tracheal line in the case of an aneurysm involving the aortic arch;
- Abnormal lateralization of the left para-spinal line in the case of an aneurysm involving the descending thoracic aorta [1].

The diagnostic process may be facilitated if a linear calcific area is identified in the context of a mediastinal area of radiopacity adjacent to the aorta, corresponding to an intimal calcification delimiting the aneurysmal profile [2]. However, this finding does not always correspond to an intimal calcification, but may instead be determined by a calcification of the false lumen; this leads to the necessity of a differential diagnosis between aortic dissection and partially calcified thoracic aortic aneurysm [3].

It is not possible to correctly measure the width of the aneurysm on chest X-ray images, because of the frequent magnification artifacts' presence; in addition to that, the edges of the artery are not always well visualized.

The differential diagnosis includes mediastinal masses that may deflect vascular structures, resulting in an enlargement of the area of radiopacity corresponding to them [2].

Small sack-like aneurysms of the aortic arch may present on chest X-ray with an "iceberg" image, apparently separated from aorta; this leads to an harder differential diagnosis with mediastinal masses, necessarily requiring an in-depth examination with a second-level instrumental examination (chest CT).

Aneurysms originating from the inferior aortic arch's surface can be detected on chest radiogram only when partially calcified or whether a pulmonary interface is present (Fig. 7.1). Alternatively, aneurysms of this vascular portion may cause

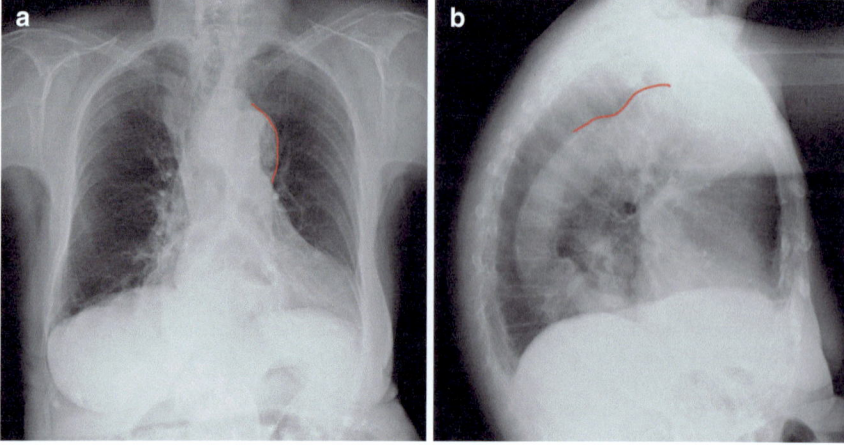

Fig. 7.1 Chest X-ray in PA projection (**a**) and in LL projection (**b**). Red: profile of the aneurysm of the ascending thoracic aorta, whose wall appears partially calcified

compression on the left main bronchus, resulting in lung parenchymal atelectasis, visible as an area of parenchymal radiopacity. This can be assumed as an indirect indicator of vascular pathology [4].

Aortic Dissection

This pathology presents with the following relatively nonspecific radiological findings, which must be clinically correlated to reach an early diagnosis:

- Mediastinal enlargement: >8 cm, at the level of the second mediastinal arch in a supine projection, >6 cm in an orthostatic one [5]. Obviously, on a first examination of chest radiogram, acquisition errors must have been excluded, since these may result in an apparent dimensional increase of the mediastinum [6]. However, mediastinal widening as a radiographic finding is more useful in the discrimination of type A aortic dissections (involving the ascending aorta or the aortic arch), since it is less frequent in type B dissections (involving the descending aorta, downstream of the emergence of the epiaortic vessels) [5].
- Double aortic contour.
- Different diameter between ascending and descending aorta [7]. Irregularity of the aortic margin, which may appear blurred ("blurring") or enlarged [8].
- Atherosclerotic calcification of the aorta in an abnormal position (distance from the aortic arch >1 cm) [7, 9]. This finding is highly suggestive of pathology but is present in a minority of cases [8].

Mediastinal widening and double aortic contour are the most frequent findings on chest X-ray in subjects with aortic dissection (>90%) [7]; therefore, if detected, they are highly indicative for the suspected pathology (Figs. 7.2 and 7.3).

The differential diagnosis includes thoracic aortic aneurysm, since enlargement of the second mediastinal arch is also evident in this case.

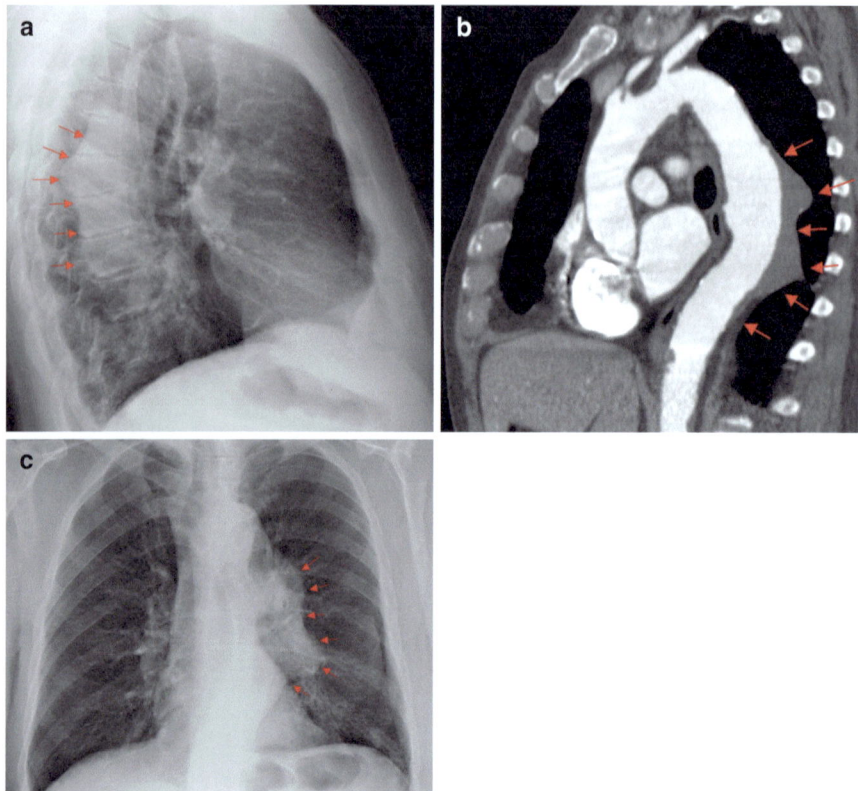

Fig. 7.2 (**a**) Magnification and deformation of the posterior profile of the descending thoracic aorta in the latero-lateral projection on chest Rx. (**b**) Magnification and deformation of the para-aortic line in the postero-anterior projection on chest Rx. (**c**) Sagittal angio-CT reconstruction of the same patient showing bilobed aneurysm of the descending thoracic aorta, with parietal thrombotic apposition

7 Abnormal Findings

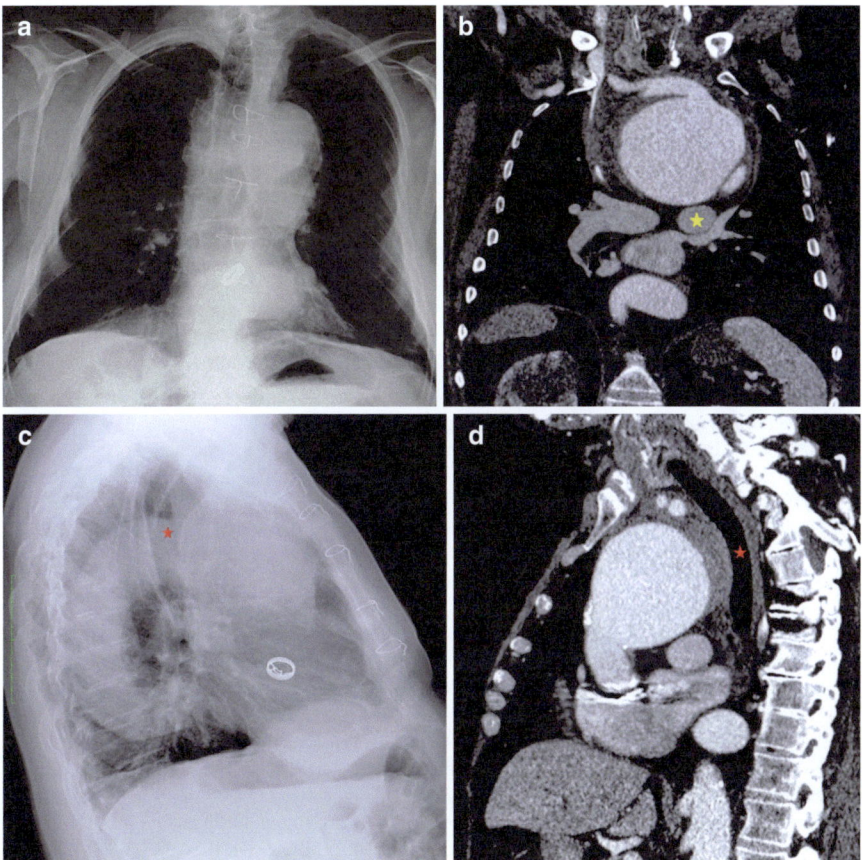

Fig. 7.3 Patient with previous aortic dissection type A surgically treated, with aneurysmal evolution of the distal ascending aorta and proximal aortic arch dissection. In (**a**) we appreciate the severe dimensional increase of the left superior cardiac arch, the obliteration of the aorto-pulmonary space and the downward displacement of the left II cardiac arch, corresponding to the left pulmonary trunk-pulmonary artery (yellow star in **b**). On latero-lateral chest Rx (**c**) and sagittal reconstruction of CT angiography (**d**), the trachea's middle III (red star) is posteriorly dislocated by the aneurysmatic distal ascending aorta-proximal aortic arch

Mediastinal or Para-Tracheal Hematoma

Consequent to aortic dissection, we can observe radiographic findings that suggest a mediastinal or para-tracheal hematoma:

- Indistinct or obscured aortic arch [10];
- deviation of mediastinal structures:
- esophagus (or naso-gastric tube) dislocated on the right side,

- trachea's dislocation on the right side,
- Increased thickness of the right and/or left para-tracheal lines (with loss of the aorto-pulmonary space) [1];
- opacification of the pulmonary apices, particularly on the left side.

Warning. A normal chest X-ray may falsely reassure the clinician! If the patient's signs and symptoms suggest an acute aortic syndrome, CT angiography should be performed immediately.

References

1. Gibbs JM, Chandrasekhar CA, Ferguson EC, et al. Lines and stripes: where did they go? From conventional radiography to CT. Radiographics. 2007;27(1):33–48.
2. Wixson D, Baltaxe HA. Pitfalls in the plain film evaluation of the thoracic aorta: the mimicry of aneurysms and adjacent masses and the value of aortography. Cardiovasc Radiol. 1979;2(2):69–76.
3. Hachiya J, Nitatori T. Calcified false channel wall in aortic dissection. Nihon Igaku Hoshasen Gakkai Zasshi. 1994;54(4):258–63.
4. Kulkarni TP, Ghandi MJ. The syndrome of compression of the pulmonary artery by an aneurysm of the ascending aorta. A case report. Am Heart J. 1963;65(5):678–82.
5. Lai V, Tsang WK, Chan WC, et al. Diagnostic accuracy of mediastinal width measurement on posteroanterior and anteroposterior chest radiographs in the depiction of acute nontraumatic thoracic aortic dissection. Emerg Radiol. 2012;19(4):309–15.
6. Gleeson CE, Spedding RL, Harding LA, et al. The mediastinum—is it wide? Emerg Med J. 2001;18(3):183–5.
7. Klompas M. Does this patient have an acute thoracic aortic dissection? The rational clinical examination. JAMA. 2002;287(17):2262–72.
8. Slater EE, DeSanctis RW. The clinical recognition of dissecting aortic aneurysm. Am J Med. 1976;60(5):625–33. https://doi.org/10.1016/0002-9343(76)90496-4. ISSN 0002-9343. PMID: 1020750.
9. Gartland S, Sookur D, Lee H. Aortic dissection: an x ray sign. Emerg Med J. 2007;24(4):310.
10. Stark P, Cook M. Traumatic rupture of the thoracic aorta. A review of 49 cases. Radiologe. 1987;27(9):402–6.

Part III

Aortic Aneurysms: Pre-treatment Evaluation

Thoracic Aortic Diseases

8

Pier Giorgio Nardis, Bianca Rocco, Simone Ciaglia, Mario Corona, Simone Zilahi de Gyurgyokai, and Carlo Catalano

Introduction

Thoracic aorta aneurysm (TAA) is a pathological, progressive, dilatation at least 50% greater than the adjacent healthy portion of the vessel [1, 2]. The incidence of this pathology is 5–10 cases per 100,000.

According to the location, aneurysms can be classified into *ascending aortic aneurysms* (ATAA) (60% of cases) and *descending aortic aneurysms* (DTAA) (40% of cases). In addition, 10% of ATAAs involve the aortic arch, and 10% of DTAAs are located in the *thoracoabdominal aorta* [3].

The risk of rupture or dissection for 6 cm ascending aortic aneurysm is 31%, while for 7 cm descending aortic aneurysm the risk is 43%.

Therefore, according to the Society of Thoracic Surgery, treatment is recommended when aortic aneurysms exceed 5.5 cm (in case of surgical replacement 6 cm is considered for descending aortic aneurysm) to prevent dissection or rupture. Lower threshold values (>4.5 cm for the ascending aorta and >5.5 cm for the descending aorta) are considered in patients with connective tissue disease (Marfan disease) or evidence of aneurysmal growth (>5 mm/year).

Aortic index [aortic diameter (cm)/body surface (m^2)] can be considered to determinate the risk of complication of rupture (2.75 cm/m^2 correlated to 8% annual risk of rupture) [4] in brachytype.

Moreover treatment is mandatory in patients with symptoms (chest pain, imaging) of rupture regardless of aortic diameter.

P. G. Nardis (✉) · B. Rocco · S. Ciaglia · M. Corona · S. Z. de Gyurgyokai · C. Catalano
Vascular and Interventional Radiology Unit, Department of Radiological, Oncological and Anathomo-Patological Science, Policlinico Umberto I, "Sapienza" University of Rome, Rome, Italy
e-mail: p.nardis@policlinicoumberto1.it; mario.corona@uniroma1.it; carlo.catalano@uniroma1.it

Ascending Thoracic Aortic Aneurysms (ATAA)

Ascending thoracic aortic aneurysms (ATAA) are classified according to their location as:

- Aortic root aneurysms: the segment between the aortic-ventricular junction (aortic annulus) and the sinotubular junction (Fig. 8.1a);
- Tubular tract aneurysms: between the sinotubular junction and the origin of the supraortic vessels (Fig. 8.1b).

Conservative Treatment

The most recent guidelines on radiological surveillance suggest 12 months interval CT/MR follow-up for ascending aortic aneurysms <4 cm, while in patients with aneurysms between 4 cm and 5.5 cm, 6-months interval CT/MR follow-up is recommended [1, 2].

Conservative treatment includes atherosclerosis risk factors and blood pressure control in order to reduce the risk of dissections or ruptures [5].

Surgical Treatment

The gold standard for the treatment of ascending aortic aneurysms is open surgery for proximal aorta with or without the use of protection device for the brain [6].

The techniques include isolated replacement of the ascending aorta (Wheat's surgery, Fig. 8.2a) or a complete aortic root replacement (Bentall's surgery, Fig. 8.2b) with or without aortic arch replacement [7].

In young patients with aortic root aneurysm, the valve can be replaced using the patient's own pulmonary valve (Ross surgery) (Fig. 8.2c). The pulmonary valve is then replaced with a biological or synthetic prosthesis. The advantages of the Ross operation include hemodynamics improvements, lower risk of endocarditis, and lower thrombogenicity [8].

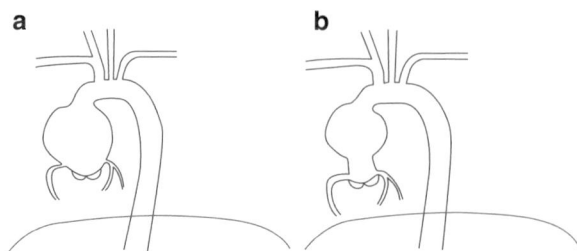

Fig. 8.1 Classification of AATA: (**a**) aortic root aneurysms, (**b**) ascending tract aneurysms

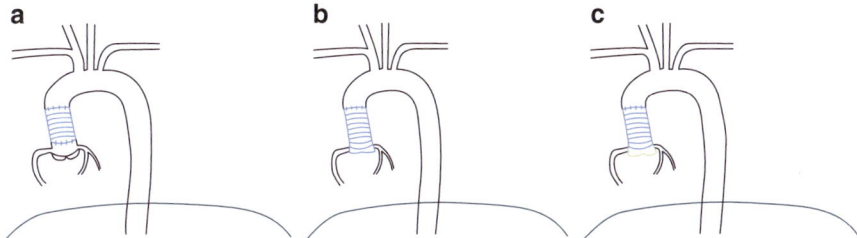

Fig. 8.2 (**a**) Wheat technique: the prosthesis of the ascending aorta is placed distal to the coronary ostium. (**b**) Bentall technique: the aortic root is replaced by a prosthesis with an integrated aortic valve and anastomosis of the coronary arteries. (**c**) Ross "valve-sparing" technique: the native aorta is replaced with Dacron prosthesis and the aortic valve with pulmonary valve (yellow)

Post-Surgical Imaging

Even if ultrasound can be considered for preliminary evaluation, CT represents the main tool for post-operative imaging findings. Small amount of fluid or air bubble can be observed in the immediate post-operative period as post-surgical changes but it generally reduces in few days. Infections have to be suspected if large amount of fluid with air bubbles persist and increase over time, together with post-contrast enhancement of periprosthetic soft tissue.

Infections are generally due to aerobic bacteria; large amount of air in the mediastinum can indicate fistula with an adjacent bronchus or esophagus.

Synthetic prostheses are commonly composed of polyethylene (Dacron) and are slightly hyperdense compared to the native aortic wall on unenhanced CT.

Although prosthesis can be barely seen on contrast CT scan, its position can usually be determined by the abrupt change in contour between the graft and native aorta or by visualizing high-attenuation felt rings Teflon made [8]. Due to the hyperdensity of the "webbing," it can be misinterpreted as pathological finding (pseudoaneurysms) on arterial phase CT scans; the unenhanced scans, thanks to their hyperdensity, allow the correct diagnosis. Moreover, potential complications of ascending aortic repairs include anastomotic pseudoaneurysm and hemorrhage.

Pseudoaneurysms can be classified into infected and non-infected:

- Infected pseudoaneurysms can be saccular with narrow neck, irregular border associated with inflammatory stranding. Their growth can be fast with an increased risk of rupture.
- Non-infected pseudoaneurysm showed a regular border, slow growing, and no inflammatory stranding is observed.

Hemorrhagic changes can be seen as a hyperattenuation area (>30 HU) adjacent to the graft or at the access site. Potential mimics in this case could be post-operative blood, calcium or reinforcement material but generally contrast media extravasation can allow to the correct diagnosis [9].

Aortic Arch Aneurysms

Aortic arch aneurysms are generally associated with aneurysms of the ascending or descending aorta. The criteria to consider aneurysm dilatation of the aortic arch are the same described for the ascending aortic aneurysm (diameter >50% of the adjacent healthy part of the vessel). The incidence and natural evolution of disease are still relatively unknown.

Surgical Treatment

According to the 2010 American Heart Association guidelines for surgical treatment of aortic arch aneurysms [1, 2], surgical replacement is indicated for acute aortic dissections with rupture or extensive involvement of supraortic vessel, whole aortic arch aneurysms, and chronic dissection associated with arch aneurysm.

Open Standard Technique

The open standard technique consists in replacement of the aortic arch with a prosthesis with or without branching of the epiaortic vessels.

For distal arch aneurysms that also involve the proximal descending thoracic aorta, whole arch replacement with elephant trunk technique is usually preferred [10]. The elephant trunk is performed in two steps to reduce the risk of intraoperative aortic rupture. In the first step a prosthesis is placed at the level of the ascending, arch and descending proximal aorta (Fig. 8.3a, b) and supraortic vessels are anastomized to the graft [11]. At the end of the first stage, the distal end of the aortic prosthesis remains free in the descending aorta. Some days later a second graft is

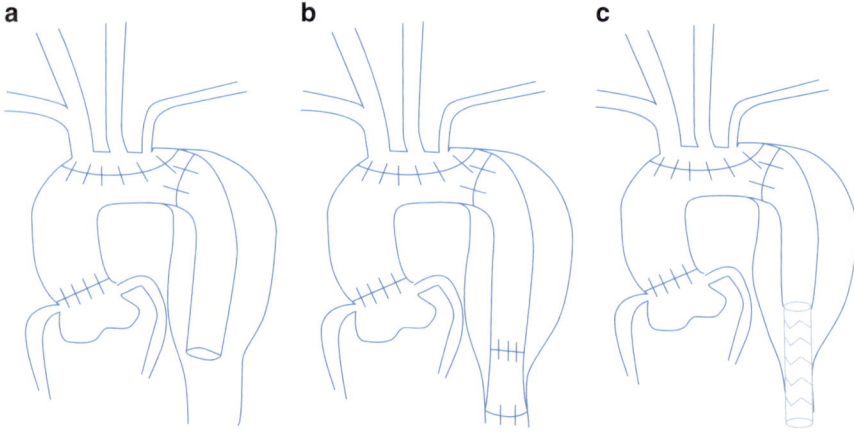

Fig. 8.3 Elephant trunk technique in arch and descending thoracic aorta aneurysm: (**a**) Replacement of ascending aorta and arch with surgical prosthesis beating into descending thoracic aorta; (**b**) Packing of distal surgical prosthesis anastomosed with distal collar of aneurysm. (**c**) Endovascular completion with endoprosthesis

placed in the descending aorta or in the thoracoabdominal aorta and connected to the prosthesis previously implanted. Alternatively, the second stage can be completed by placing an endograft (hybrid elephant trunk) (Fig. 8.3c).

Endovascular Techniques

Thoracic endovascular aortic repair (TEVAR) can be considered in the treatment of ascending aortic and aortic arch pathologies together with open surgery in patients unfit for surgery.

The most common surgical-endovascular hybrid approach in the treatment of ascending aorta and aortic arch pathologies consists of endovascular exclusion with stent-graft together with debranching of the epiaortic vessels [12].

According to the location of the aneurysm and consequently the landing zone of the stent-graft, debranching can be performed using different techniques:

1. sequential by-pass between epiaortic vessels (carotid-carotid-subclavian by-pass) in order to gain proximal aortic neck if the aneurysm involves the distal part of the aortic arch (Fig. 8.4);
2. total debranching of the epiaortic vessel using a multi-branched graft between the ascending aorta and the epiaortic vessels [13] (Fig. 8.5).

Fig. 8.4 Scheme of supraortic vessel revascularization in case of endovascular repair of aortic arch aneurysm

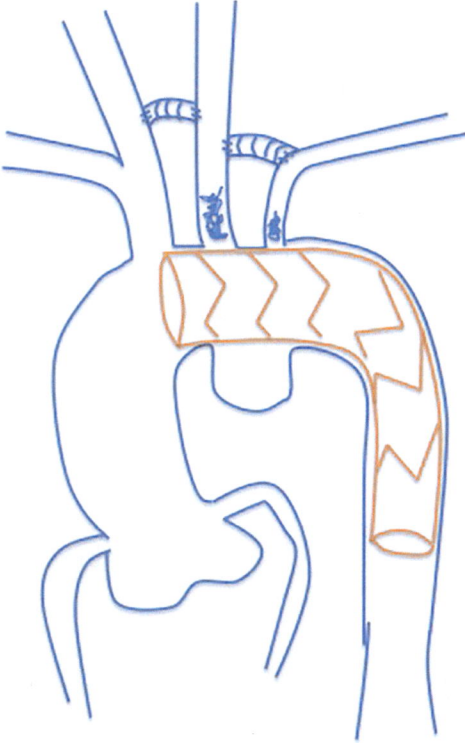

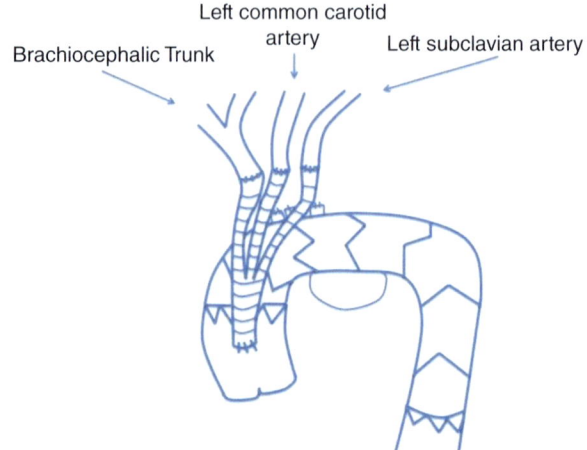

Fig. 8.5 Total debranching of the epiaortic vessel using a multi branched graft

Due to the increasing use of endovascular techniques, some centers have described the use of latest generation branched or fenestrated endoprosthesis or chimney technique, with good technical success and low perioperative morbidity and mortality.

It consists of fenestrated or branched stent-graft that allow fully endovascular treatment of ascending and aortic arch pathologies in patients unfit for surgery (Figs. 8.6a, b and 8.7); however, there are few reports and data on this treatment and it has to be considered in selected case and multicenter randomized trials, data on efficacy and long-term durability are still lacking [14].

Some authors described the Chimney and Periscope technique (for details about Chimney and Periscope Technique see Chap. 10) as an alternative endovascular option for aortic arch aneurysm with short proximal neck, in patients unfit for surgery (Fig. 8.6c). It consists of endovascular exclusion of aortic arch-descending aortic pathologies together with parallel stent-graft in the epiaortic vessels according to the location of the disease. Despite the feasibility of this technique, the incidence of type I endoleak (gutter endoleak) is very high due to the poor adhesion of the stent-graft to the vessel wall; for this reason, this option is considered in selected cases generally in emergency settings.

8 Thoracic Aortic Diseases

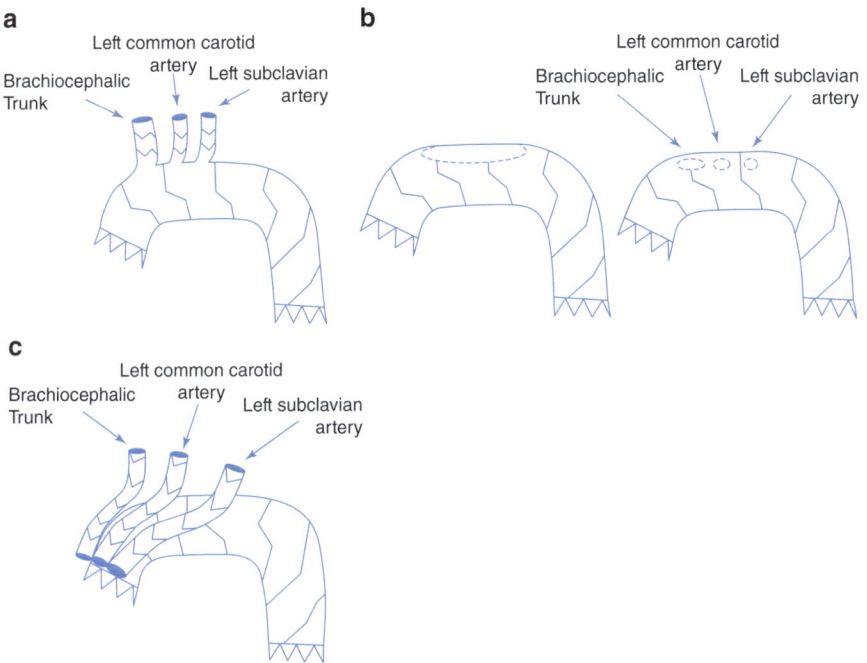

Fig. 8.6 (**a–c**) Different endovascular techniques for the treatment of the arch's pathologies. (**a**) Multibranched endoprosthesis (**b**) fenestrated endoprosthesis (**c**) chimney technique

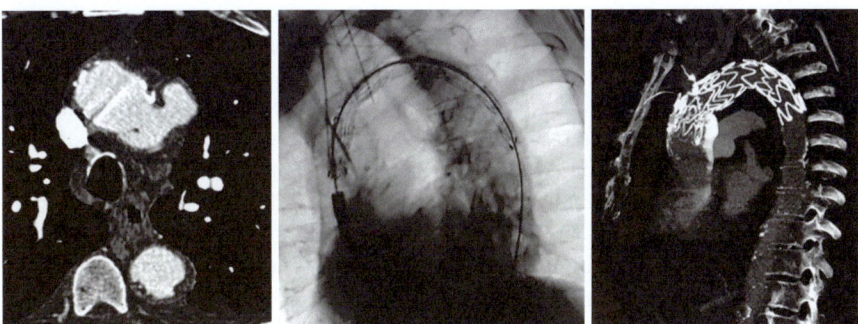

Fig. 8.7 Sacciform aneurysm of the aortic arch treated by implantation of custom endoprosthesis with fenestration for the epiaortic vessels

Aneurysms of the Descending Thoracic Aorta (DTAA) and Acute (descending) Aortic Syndrome

The treatment of descending thoracic aorta has been redefined with the development of thoracic endovascular aneurysm repair (TEVAR). TEVAR should be considered the treatment of choice when DTAA diameter is greater than 55 mm. Lower threshold should be considered in patients with Marfan syndrome or other elastopathies [15].

DTAAs are classified, according to the Safi's classification [1, 2], into:

- *Type A*: involving the proximal portion of the descending aorta, with extension from the left subclavian artery to the sixth rib;
- *Type B*: involving the distal portion of the descending aorta, from the sixth rib to the diaphragmatic hiatus;
- *Type C*: involving the tract from the subclavian to the diaphragmatic hiatus.

Acute (descending) aortic syndromes include aortic dissection, intramural hematoma, and penetrating atherosclerotic ulcer (PAU). They share clinical manifestations such as intense chest pain or back pain with sudden onset that usually can be extended to the abdomen or pelvis. In classical spontaneous aortic dissection, blood pressure separates the aortic wall layers from an initiating intimal tear and generates a false lumen. False lumen blood pressure is higher compared to the true lumen, leading to a compression of the true lumen with possible rupture or malperfusion syndrome. Intramural hematoma can be appreciated in non-contrast CT scan as hyperattenuating focal, elongated or circumferential area. PAU is a disease of the intimal layer with a background of atherosclerotic disease with progressive penetration on the ulcer through the aortic wall with eventual rupture or dissection. PAU is distinguished from a common ulcerated plaque because it reaches the medial layer and it is often associated with symptoms and can be quickly recognized as an hemorrhage in the medial layer, often associated with thrombus. Stanford and DeBakey classification systems are based on anatomic lesion site and extension. The Stanford classification is most widely used for its simplicity in aiding in decision making on acute phases [16].

Acute traumatic aortic injuries (ATAI) vary widely from intimal tear to complete transection. Rapid deceleration in antero-posterior or lateral directions are often sufficient to have a cardiac displacement and, consequently, torsion and shearing force to the aorta at the level of ligamentum arteriosum, aortic root, and diaphragm. CT scan is the imaging of choice for diagnosis of ATAI thanks to its fast acquisition and high diagnostic sensitivity (Fig. 8.8). Indirect findings consist of mediastinal hematoma while direct findings are the presence of intimal flap, traumatic pseudoaneurysm, contained rupture, abnormal aortic contour, and sudden change in aortic caliber. The aortic isthmus is the most common location for ATAI due to its relative fixed position, within the thorax and connected to ligamentum arteriosum [17]. More details on diagnostic imaging of acute aortic syndrome and rupture will be widely discussed in Chap. 5.

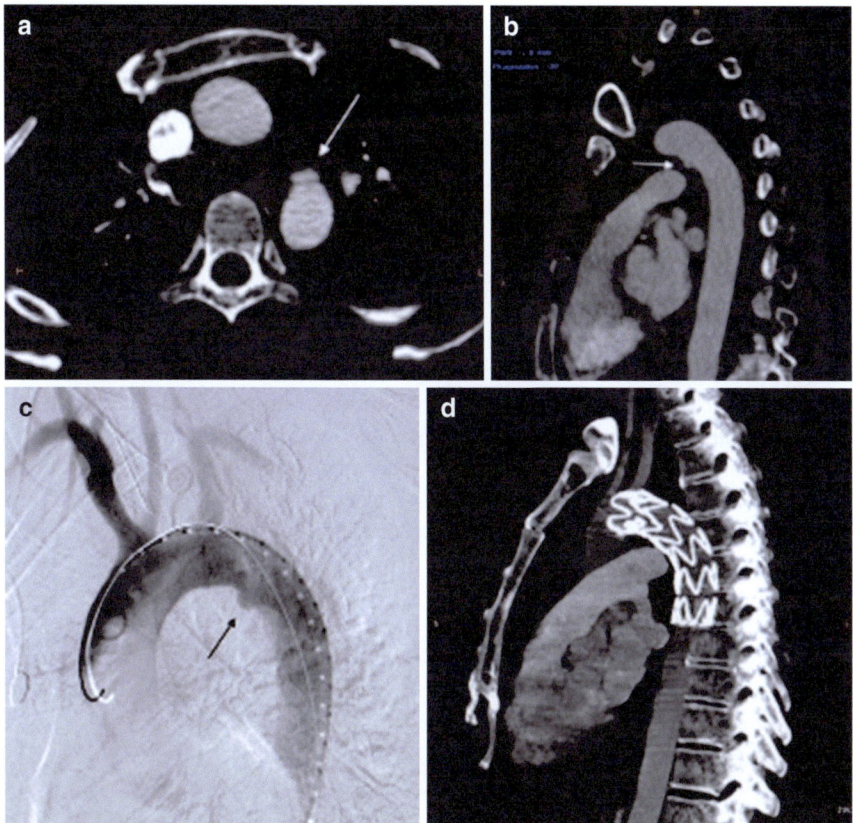

Fig. 8.8 CT images of a young patient involved in a car accident showed pseudoaneurysm of the descending thoracic aorta (**a**, **b**). Angiography performed during TEVAR confirmed pseudoaneurysm (**c**), 1-month CT follow-up (**d**)

Surgical Treatment

The current surgery for treating DTAA was described by Crawford in 1974. The technique consists in aneurysm section or aortic prosthesis placement to repair the aneurysmal aortic tract, followed by reimplantation of visceral vessels and intercostal arteries to the aortic prosthesis to minimize the risk of paraplegia. Due to the increased risk of paraplegia, even with short aortic clamping times (risk of 27% after 60 min and 8% after 30 min), nowadays the clamp-and-sew technique is abandoned. Intraoperative innovations has been introduced such as aortic perfusion during aortic clamping, moderate systemic hypothermia at 33–34 °C, cerebrospinal fluid (CSF) drainage and reimplantation of intercostal arteries [5].

Endovascular Treatment

Endovascular treatment of DTAAs (TEVAR), initially proposed for patients not suitable for open surgery [6], has shown promising results since its introduction in 1994 and in 2005 was approved by the Food and Drug Administration (FDA). Currently, TEVAR has been recommended as first-line treatment for elective and urgent DTAAs or as bridging to open surgery in case of patients with connective tissue disease. The development of new materials, manufacturing, device delivery systems, and the operator experience has allowed an increase of indications. TEVAR has replaced open surgery in most cases of thoracic descending aortic diseases, due to reduced peri-procedural morbidity and mortality (Fig. 8.9a–f). TEVAR is now also approved for the treatment of complicated type B aortic dissection with malperfusion syndrome, rupture, traumatic aortic injuries, and penetrating aortic ulcers. All devices are generally made of nitinol stents covered by polytetrafluoroethylene (e-PTFE) aiming to exclude the diseased tract (aneurysm, PAU, intramural hematoma, dissection) from the bloodstream. As weel as in thoracic aortic aneurysm, penetrating atherosclerotic ulcer, thoracic aortic traumatic rupture and intramural

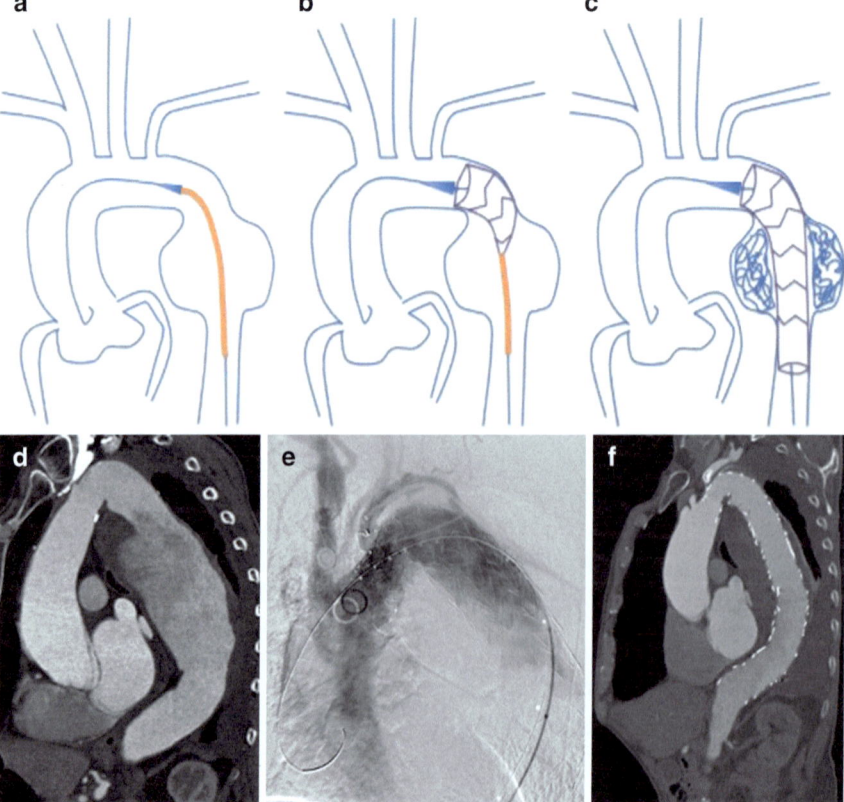

Fig. 8.9 (**a–c**) TEVAR scheme for AATD; (**d–f**) fusiform descending thoracic aortic aneurysm treated with endoprosthesis

8 Thoracic Aortic Diseases

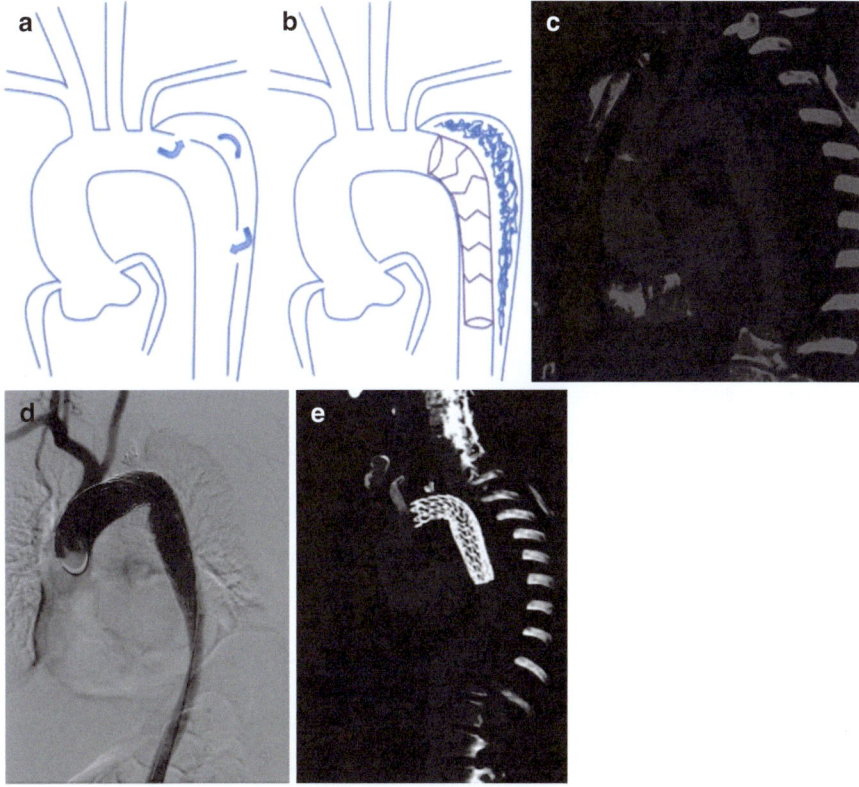

Fig. 8.10 TEVAR in the treatment of type B aortic dissection

hematoma, the aim is to exclude the diseased aortic tract from the bloodstream, the purpose of treatment in aortic dissection is covering intimal tear by placing a stent-graft in the true lumen in order to reduce blood flow and pressure in the false lumen, and promote thrombosis (Fig. 8.10a–e).

Pretreatment CT Scan Evaluation

Proximal Neck and Distal Neck

The proximal and distal neck are the keypoint for the outcome of endovascular treatment of a thoracic aneurysm or dissection; they represent the segment of healthy aorta upstream and downstream of the diseased tract where the stent-graft will be fixed. The characteristics of the neck are length and diameter.

1. *Length*: As a general rule, in a relatively straight descending thoracic aorta, a proximal and distal neck length of 2 cm is usually adequate as landing zone for

an endoprosthesis, allowing adequate sealing; in case of tortuous anatomy and in those aneurysms of the proximal descending thoracic aorta or type B dissection, close to the curve of the aortic arch, a longer proximal neck is required to allow endoprosthesis conformation and vessel wall adhesion. In cases of short proximal neck, left subclavian artery can be partially or fully covered by the stent-graft in order to obtain greater anchorage; further surgical revascularization can be performed (Fig. 8.11) before or after the endovascular treatment. Revascularization of the left subclavian artery is generally performed in elective surgery, while in emergency settings, it can be avoided or postponed thanks to the good collateralization of the axillary artery. Although in some centers left subclavian artery revascularization is not routinely performed even in elective cases, recent studies have revealed a higher risk of arm ischemia and vertebro-basilar ischemia compared to patients in which preoperative revascularization has been performed.
2. *Diameter*: An adequate information on the caliber of the neck is crucial because the endoprosthesis correctly adheres to the vessel wall due to its radial force. The ideal caliber of a stent-graft to achieve a perfect adhesion to the aortic wall, should be 10–20% larger than the diameter of the aortic neck (e.g., aortic neck caliber of 20 mm, endoprosthesis caliber of 22–24 mm). An undersized endo-

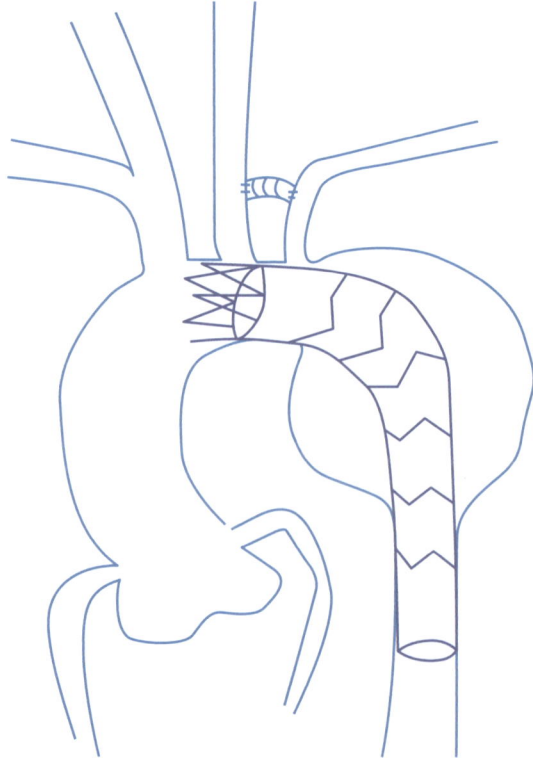

Fig. 8.11 Scheme of endovascular exclusion of thoracic aortic aneurysm with subclavian artery occlusion; carotid-subclavian bypass was performed for the subclavian revascularization

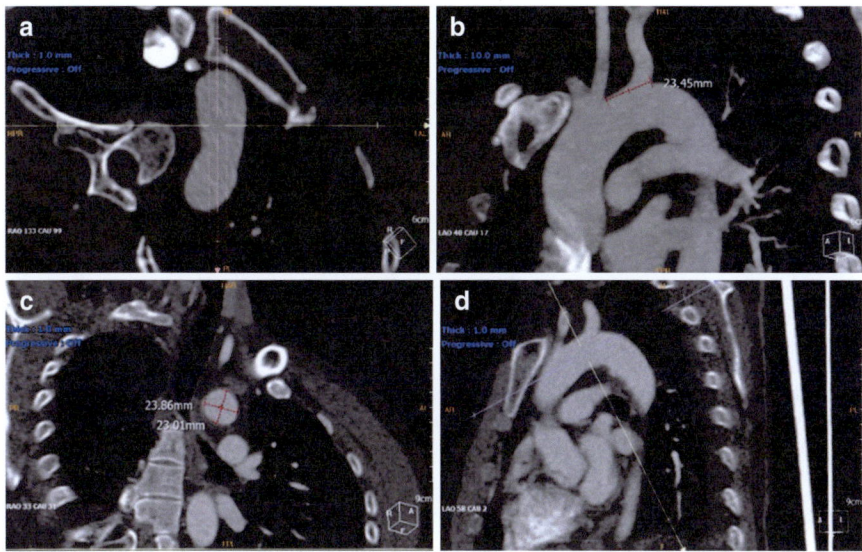

Fig. 8.12 MPR or curved reconstruction for the evaluation of the aortic neck is useful to give the most proper information (**a, b, c, d**)

prosthesis could lead to some complications such as a risk for dislocation and endoleak, while an oversized endoprosthesis could lead to an infolding of the graft. In case of aortic dissection the aortic caliber to be considered includes true and false lumen together (median-median layer).

Both the length and the diameter of the neck have to be evaluated using MPR or curved reconstructions, or using vessel analysis protocol, in order to give the most proper information (Fig. 8.12).

Anatomy of the Aortic Arch and Origin of the Epiaortic Vessels

The anatomy of the aortic arch is crucial for thoracic endoprosthesis implantation because it affects in some cases the proximal landing site of the endoprosthesis (e.g., aortic aneurysm involves the proximal descending thoracic aorta or this tract can be used as a healthy vessel to treat the proximal intimal dissection located near the origin of the left subclavian artery).

Angulation of the arch represents a key point in the implantation of an endoprosthesis: as the angle of aortic arch increases the more difficulties of stent-graft implantation will be. As shown in Fig. 8.13, there are three types of arch, depending on the origin of the anonymous trunk in relation to a plane lying on the upper profile of the aortic arch.

The origin of the supraortic vessel is another keypoint in the planning of endovascular treatment. Figure 8.14 shows some examples of the most frequently

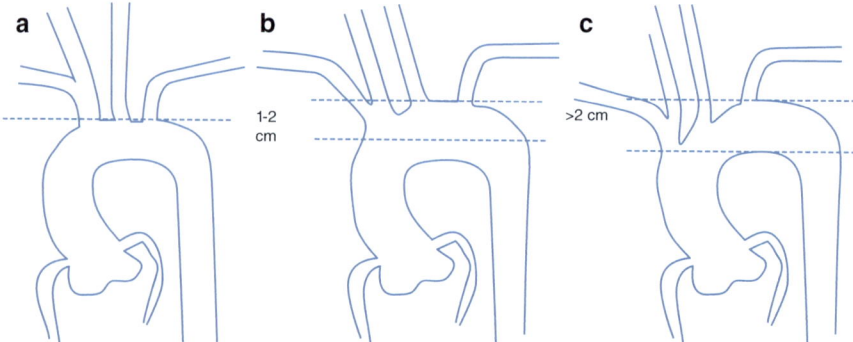

Fig. 8.13 Summary diagram showing the various types of aortic arch. Aortic arch can be divide into three types according the distance between the innominate artery and a horizontal line through the top of arch: (**a**) Type 1—less than 1 cm; (**b**) Type 2—between 1 and 2 cm; (**c**) Type 3—more than 3 cm

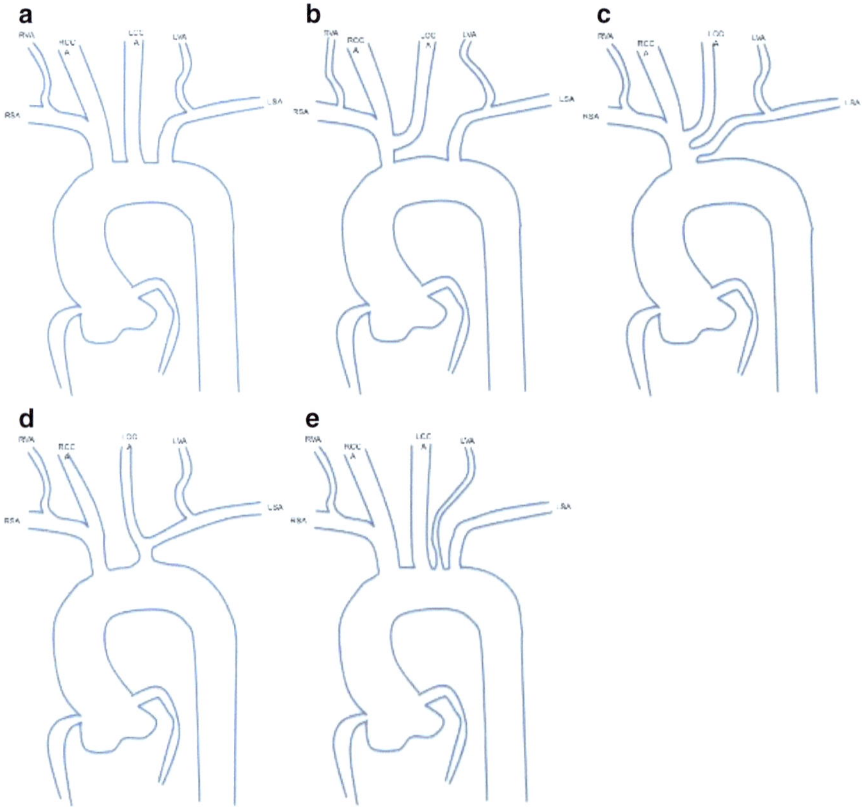

Fig. 8.14 (**a**) Normal anatomy; (**b**) bovine arch; (**c**) common epiaortic trunk; (**d**) common subclavian artery and left common carotid artery origin; (**e**) isolated origin from the aortic arch of the left vertebral artery

anatomical variants. To give an example, a common epiaortic trunk (Fig. 8.14c) is a favorable condition, while the presence of a left brachiocephalic trunk (Fig. 8.14d) with common origin of the subclavian and the left carotid arteries, in case of a short neck of the aneurysm, is an unfavorable condition requiring surgical revascularization of left carotid artery before endovascular treatment.

Intercostal Arteries

As mentioned before, the risk of spinal cord ischemia and paraplegia depends on occlusion of spinal arteries that arise from intercostal arteries at the level of descending thoracic aorta, by the stent-graft. Consequently, in order to reduce the risk of this catastrophic complication, large intercostal arteries have to be identified and reported so that the interventionalist can save during the procedure as much as possible.

References

1. Hiratzka LF, Bakris GL, Beckman JA, et al. ACCF/AHA/AATS/ACR/ASA/SCA/SCAI/SIR/STS/SVM guidelines for the diagnosis and management of patients with thoracic aortic disease. A report of the American College of Cardiology Foundation/American Heart Association task force on practice guidelines, American Association for Thoracic Surgery, American College of Radiology, American Stroke Association, Society of Cardio-vascular Anesthesiologists, Society for Cardiovascular Angiography and Interventions, Society of Interventional Radiology, Society of Thoracic Surgeons and Society for Vascular Medicine. J Am Coll Cardiol. 2010a;55(14):e27–e129.
2. Hiratzka LF, Bakris GL, Beckman JA, Bersin RM, Carr VF, Casey DE, Eagle KA, Hermann LK, Isselbacher EM, Kazerooni EA, Kouchoukos NT, Lytle BW, Milewicz DM, Reich DL, Sen S, Shinn JA, Svensson LG, Williams DM, American College of Cardiology Foundation, American Heart Association Task Force on Practice Guidelines, American Association for Thoracic Surgery, American College of Radiology, American Stroke Association, Society of Cardiovascular Anesthesiologists, Society for Cardiovascular Angiography and Interventions, Society of Interventional Radiology, Society of Thoracic Surgeons, Society for Vascular Medicine. 2010 ACCF/AHA/AATS/ACR/ASA/SCA/SCAI/SIR/STS/SVM guidelines for the diagnosis and management of patients with thoracic aortic disease: executive summary. A report of the American College of Cardiology Foundation/American Heart Association task force on practice guidelines, American Association for Thoracic Surgery, American College of Radiology, American Stroke Association, Society of Cardiovascular Anesthesiologists, Society for Cardiovascular Angiography and Interventions, Society of Interventional Radiology, Society of Thoracic Surgeons, and Society for Vascular Medicine. Catheter Cardiovasc Interv. 2010b;76(2):E43–86.
3. Kuzmik GA, Sang AX, Elefteriades JA. Natural history of thoracic aortic aneurysms. J Vasc Surg. 2012;56(2):565–71.
4. Svensson LG, Kouchoukos NT, Miller DC, et al. Expert consensus document on the treatment of descending thoracic aortic disease using endovascular stent-grafts. Ann Thorac Surg. 2008;85(1):S1–41.
5. Goldfinger JZ, Halperin JL, Marin ML, et al. Thoracic aortic aneurysm and dissection. J Am Coll Cardiol. 2014;64(16):1725–39.
6. Jain D, Dietz HC, Oswald GL, et al. Causes and histopathology of ascending aortic disease in children and young adults. Cardiovasc Pathol. 2011;20(1):15–25.

7. Elefteriades JA, Ziganshin BA, Rizzo JA, et al. Indications and imaging for aortic surgery: size and other matters. J Thorac Cardiovasc Surg. 2015;149:S10–3.
8. Hoang JK, Martinez S, Hurwitz LM. MDCT angiography after open thoracic aortic surgery: pearls and pitfalls. AJR Am J Roentgenol. 2009;192(1):W20–7.
9. Marquis MK, Naeem M, Rajput ZM, Raptis DA, Steinbrecher KL, Ohman JW, Bhalla S, Rapts AC. CT of postoperative repair of the ascending aorta and aortic arch. Radiographics. 2021;41:1300–20.
10. Al Kindi AH, Al Kimyani N, Alameddine T, et al. "Open" approach to aortic arch aneurysm repair. J Saudi Heart Assoc. 2014;26(3):152–61.
11. Azizzadeh A, Estrera AL, Porat EE, et al. The hybrid elephant trunk procedure: a single-stage repair of an ascending, arch, and descending thoracic aortic aneurysm. J Vasc Surg. 2006;4(2):404–7.
12. Xydas S, Mihos CG, Williams RF, et al. Hybrid repair of aortic arch aneurysms: a comprehensive review. J Thorac Dis. 2017;9(Suppl 7):S629–34.
13. Swerdlow NJ, Wu WW, Schermerhorn ML. Open and endovascular management of aortic aneurysms. Circ Res. 2019;124(4):647–61.
14. Fiorucci B, Banafsche R, Jerkku T, et al. Thoracic aortic aneurysms—diagnosis and treatment strategies. Dtsch Med Wochenschr. 2019;144(3):146–51.
15. ESC. Guidelines on the diagnosis and treatment of aortic disease. Eur Heart J. 2014;35: 2873–926. https://doi.org/10.1093/eurheartj/ehu281.
16. Maurillo H, Molvin L, Chin SA, Fleischmann D. Aortic dissection and other acute aortic syndromes: diagnostic imaging findings from acute to chronic longitudinal progression. Radiographics. 2021;41(2):425–46.
17. Steenburg SD, Ravenel JG, Ikonomidis JS, Schönholz C, Reeves S. Acute traumatic aortic injury: imaging evaluation and management. Radiology. 2008;248(3):748–62.

Thoracoabdominal Aortic Aneurysm (Classification, CT Aspects, Pre-Procedure Evaluation, Endovascular Treatment)

Ciro Ferrer

Aortic aneurysm is defined as a localized and permanent dilatation of the aorta, with an increase in diameter of at least 50% over normal.

Thoracoabdominal aortic aneurysms result from continuous dilation of the descending thoracic aorta extending into the abdominal aorta. The classification of TAAA was developed by Crawford in 1986 [1], and then subsequently modified, and is subdivided as follows (Fig. 9.1):

- Type I: from the origin of the left subclavian artery to the suprarenal aorta;
- Type II: from the origin of the left subclavian artery to the infrarenal aorta, sometimes with involvement of the common iliac arteries;
- Type III: from the sixth intercostal space to the infrarenal aorta;
- Type IV: from the diaphragmatic hiatus to the infrarenal aorta.

The incidence of TAAAs has markedly increased over the past few decades and in the USA is around 10.4 cases per 100,000 per year [1]. The increasing incidence of TAAAs has been attributed to improved imaging methods and aging population.

The development of TAAAs is a multifactorial event involving genetic, cellular, and hemodynamic factors. The etiology of such aneurysms is predominantly related to two pathologies: atherosclerosis for 80% and aortic dissection for 15%. Other pathologies, such as Marfan syndrome and Ehlers-Danlos syndrome, or other connective tissue disorders, mycotic infections, and trauma contribute for about 5%.

C. Ferrer (✉)
Vascular and Endovascular Surgery Unit, San Giovanni-Addolorata Hospital, Rome, Italy
e-mail: cferrer@hsangiovanni.roma.it

© The Author(s), under exclusive license to Springer Nature Switzerland AG 2024
I. Carbone et al. (eds.), *Imaging of the Aorta*,
https://doi.org/10.1007/978-3-031-52527-8_9

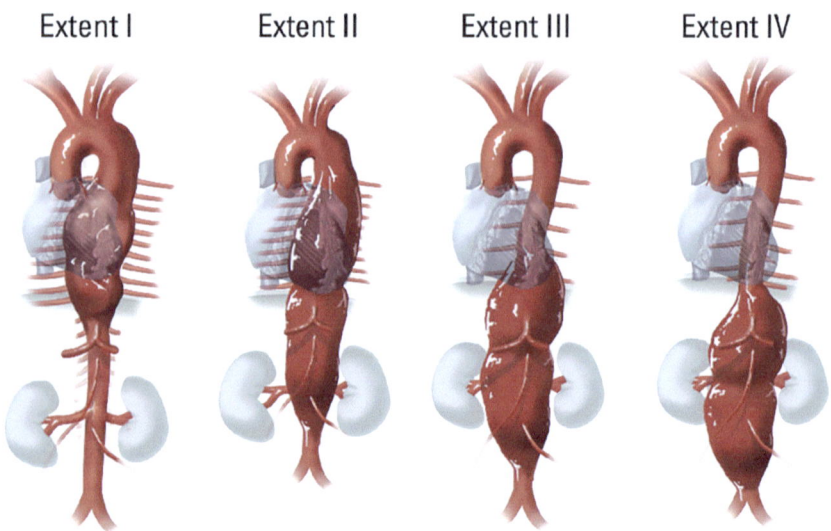

Fig. 9.1 Crawford classification of thoracoabdominal aortic aneurysms

Despite advances in surgical technique and continued improvements in the intra- and postoperative management of patients with TAAAs, traditional surgical treatment is associated with significant mortality and morbidity, primarily because of the invasiveness of surgical access and potential hemodynamic instability secondary to proximal aortic clamping and blood loss. Elective mortality rates within 5% are reported only by very high volume centers and mainly concern patients with acceptable operative risk [2]. With the progressive increase in the average age of the population and the improvement in diagnostic capabilities, an increasing number of elderly patients with multiple comorbidities and limited functional reserve are now being referred for treatment of TAAA. Hence the need to further reduce morbidity and mortality associated with traditional surgical treatment. For these reasons, the endovascular approach in the treatment of TAAAs has become a particularly attractive option today. Since the first pioneering implantation in the 1990s, endovascular exclusion of descending thoracic aortic aneurysms (TEVAR) is considered a safe alternative to open surgery and is associated with significantly lower mortality and morbidity, so that it is considered the gold standard for the treatment of isolated thoracic aneurysms [3, 4]. In the last years, the progressive refinement of endovascular techniques and the remarkable technological evolution of the devices have made it possible that also TAAAs can be treated with endovascular methods, mainly thanks to the introduction of fenestrated and branched endoprostheses. Endovascular techniques clearly guarantee less invasiveness and are associated with a lower incidence of cardiac and respiratory complications in relation to an older average age, thus allowing the treatment of patients otherwise excluded due to the high surgical risk [5]. Although data in the literature on the long-term outcomes of endovascular treatment of TAAAs are relatively limited, the advantages in terms of immediate perioperative and short-term complications compared to traditional surgery seem more than encouraging, so much so that endovascular treatment is becoming increasingly widespread [6].

The endovascular treatment of TAAA consists in the exclusion of the aneurysmal sac from the circulation, obtaining a secure attachment of the endoprosthesis proximally and distally in order to seal the aneurysmal aortic tract, ensuring the perfusion of the visceral and renal vessels with covered bridging stents connected to the aortic main body through fenestrations and/or branches. For the treatment of complex aneurysmal pathology, custom-made fenestrated (FEVAR) and branched (BEVAR) aortic endoprostheses have been developed, the latter also available in an off-the-shelf configuration. The fenestrated or branched endoprostheses consist of a main body equipped with holes (fenestrations) or channels (branches) in which covered stents necessary for the perfusion of the visceral and renal vessels are placed.

The *fenestrated endoprostheses* were born with the intent to extend the landing zone necessary to exclude AAA that do not have an infrarenal aortic neck suitable for the placement of a standard endograft (juxta- and pararenal aneurysms). In these cases, in fact, the portion of the endoprosthesis on which the fenestrations are constructed corresponds to the proximal sealing zone, which therefore by definition must be non-aneurysmal. The relatively small caliber of the aorta at this level obliges the use of fenestrations, since branches, requiring more space necessary for the correct opening, would lead to an excessive encumbrance inside the aortic lumen.

The need for *branch endoprostheses* arises from the necessity to exclude TAAA, in which by definition the portion of the paravisceral aorta is dilated and therefore usually has a larger caliber aortic lumen. This option also makes the catheterization of visceral and renal vessels easier, reducing the gap between the branch and the target vessel and giving a more anatomical conformation to the repair.

Planning and customization process requires relatively long time, from 8 to 10 weeks, sometimes incompatible with the clinical conditions of the patient. In urgent cases, alternative techniques, such as the chimney or sandwich technique, can be used. These are based on the use of standard covered stents deployed inside visceral and/or renal branches and together with the aortic main body in a parallel fashion. Greenberg was the first to describe this technique in 2003 to ensure perfusion of the visceral and renal branches during endovascular exclusion of a TAAA [7]. Multiple synonyms are commonly used to define this approach (chimney, periscope, or snorkel), all evoking the pattern of the grafts, which take the blood flow parallel to and outside the main prosthesis in order to keep patent the reno/visceral branches and ensure their perfusion, whether they originate at the proximal edge of the main aortic graft or below it, with anterograde or retrograde flow [8]. This method is potentially burdened by the high rate of endoleak through the spaces (gutters) between the covered stents, the aortic main body, and the native aorta wall, which often require additional embolization procedures that are not always resolving. In addition, the difference in radial forces between the aortic main body and visceral stents may result in compression of the latter with subsequent organ ischemia [9]. To cope with urgent and emergency situations, an off-the-shelf branched device is now available: the Cook Zenith t-Branch (Cook Medical, Bloomington, IN, USA), a thoracoabdominal endoprosthesis equipped with four branches, with a theoretical applicability of about 80% [9].

After the first case of endovascular treatment of TAAA by means of a branched endograft reported by Chuter et al. [10], several reports have been published with satisfactory results in terms of short-term mortality and morbidity. Although the vast majority of reports are based on patients treated using the Cook technology platform (Cook Medical, Bloomington, Ind, USA; Brisbane, Queensland, Australia), new models of branched or fenestrated endoprosthesis have recently been introduced, such as Jotec (Jotec GmbH, Hechingen, Germany), Anaconda, and Bolton (Terumo Aortic—Vascutek, Inchinnan, UK); however, experiences with these platforms are still limited [11].

One of the largest experiences regarding the endovascular treatment of TAAAs has been published by the Cleveland Clinic on a series of 406 patients enrolled in a prospective study with 2 years of follow-up. The perioperative mortality in this case series was 12.5% for type I, 5.2% for types II and III, and 2.3% for type IV TAAA, according to Crawford's classification. Symptoms of spinal cord ischemia (SCI) were recorded in 4.3% of cases (including 227 AAAs in addition to 406 TAAAs).

Overall survival at 2 years was 70% for type I, 74% for types II and III, and 82% for type IV TAAA [12]. Similar results were also shown by high volume European Centers [13]. Verhoeven et al. [14] described the results of 166 patients with TAAA treated with fenestrated or branched endoprostheses, reporting a mortality and perioperative SCI rate of 7.8% and 9%, respectively, and an 1-, 2-, and 5-year survival of 83%, 78%, and 66%, respectively.

The less invasive nature of the endovascular approach aims to decrease the surgical impact of traditional surgery by limiting surgical incisions, avoiding aortic clamping and subsequent intraoperative organ ischemia, reducing blood loss, hemodynamic instability, and any potential cardiac and respiratory complication. However, there is no evidence of a reduction in the incidence of what is probably one of the most serious complications of this treatment: SCI and its subsequent neurological manifestations. In addition, late complications, such as endoleaks, potential loss of stent integrity, and possible device migration, unknown for conventional treatment, may affect the long-term duration of endovascular treatment and should be balanced against the late complications and re-interventions that can potentially occur after open repair [15].

Planning

Computed tomography angiography (CTA) with its multiplanar reconstructions is the gold standard for patients with TAAA [16, 17]. By the use of workstation with dedicated software for post-processing analysis, multiplanar reconstructions according to the center lumen line (Fig. 9.2) may be useful to evaluate the suitability of the

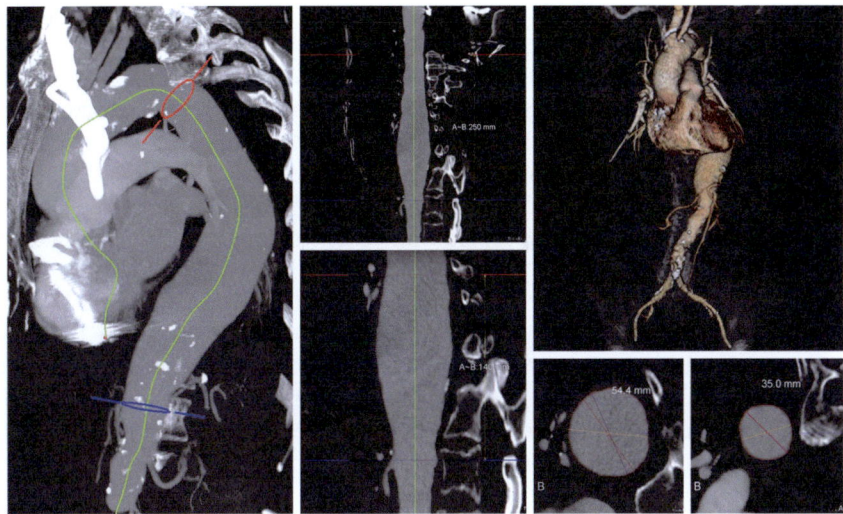

Fig. 9.2 CT multiplanar reconstruction according to the center lumen line of a type I thoracoabdominal aneurysm

landing zones, the possible presence of endoluminal thrombous, stenosis and/or tortuosity of the visceral arteries, and the quality of the access vessels, in order to determine the feasibility of the procedure and to choose the best possible configuration for the stent graft (with fenestrations, branches, or both).

When planning endovascular intervention for TAAA, the presence of an internal aortic lumen smaller than 25 mm at paravisceral/pararenal level automatically precludes the use of a branch endoprosthesis, leaving only the possibility of a custom-made fenestrated solution. Given the criteria for morphological feasibility, branched endoprostheses should be the first choice when considering endovascular treatment of TAAA. However, as in open repair, it is essential that the procedure is performed in selected Centers with appropriate technology and learning curve. Preoperative measurements are essential to design a tailored device that has the branches or fenestrations in the best position for the catheterization of the target vessels. The proximal end of the branches opens inside the main graft, while the distal end opens outside, approximately 18 mm below. In designing a branched device, each branch should be such that the distal end opens approximately 10 mm above the origin of each target vessel. While the fenestrations should be exactly calibrated at the origin of the reno-visceral vessels and oriented according to their emergence based on the clock face view, the branches may present a more liberal position in terms of axial orientation, assuming that more space is available for catheterization of the target vessels.

This explains why a standard device, with fixed position branches such as the t-Branch, is able to satisfy a wide range of applicability.

Cook T-Branch: Feasibility Assessment

Cook Medical provides a plastic model for the applicability of t-Branch which reproduces on a two-dimensional grid the three-dimensional position of the target vessels, with which the anatomical feasibility can be tested (Fig. 9.3). The steps of such a planning are shown below.

Step 1: Mark the position of the superior mesenteric artery (SMA) in the center of the grid.

Step 2: Mark the location of the celiac trunk and renal arteries on the grid.

Step 3: Mark the proximal extent of the aneurysm on the y-axis. Since the t-Branch has a fixed distance from the proximal end to the branches, the ability of the endoprosthesis to achieve proper proximal sealing will be assessed at approximately 140 mm above the origin of the SMA. The aortic diameter at this level should be between 24 and 30 mm.

Step 4: Place the plastic model in the optimal position, giving preference to the most caudal renal artery.

Step 5: Mark the level of the aortic bifurcation on the y-axis.

Step 6: Select the size of the distal bifurcated body. The bifurcated component has a fixed proximal dimension of 22 mm, while the contralateral gate opening can be chosen between 81, 98, 115, and 132 mm, depending on the level of aortic bifurcation.

Step 7: Select the iliac extensions.

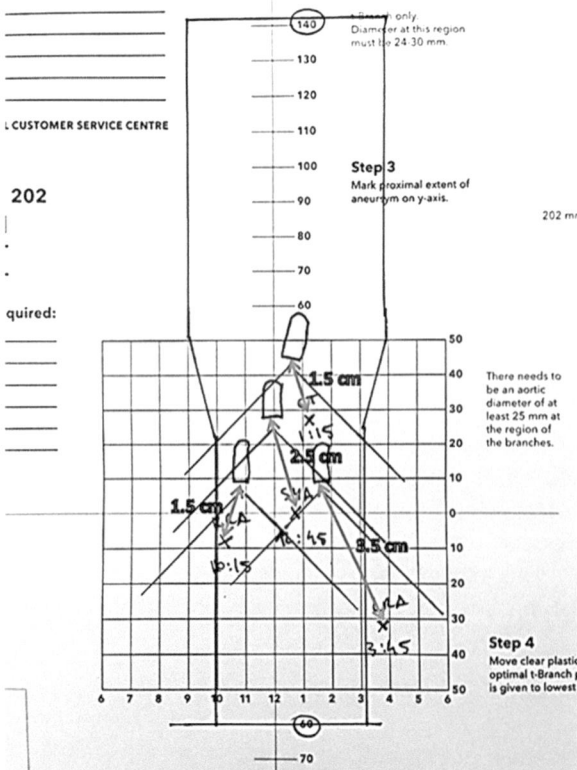

Fig. 9.3 Viscero-renal vessels spatial morphology schematic representation to assess feasibility of the off-the-shelf Cook t-Branch endoprosthesis

Procedure: Branched Endoprosthesis

With the patient under general anesthesia in supine position, with the arms along the body and the upper limbs flexed below the plane of the spine, in order to better visualize the origin of the target vessels also in lateral projection, the bilateral femoral approach is performed by surgical exposure or percutaneously using two Perclose Proglide devices (Abbott Vascular, Chicago, IL, USA) with pre-closure technique. A surgical exposure or percutaneous puncture of the axillary artery (right or left) is then performed. Alternatively, in cases where an approach from above is impossible or inadvisable, a steerable introducer sheath, inserted through a femoral access, will be used to catheterize the target vessels through the side-branches. With an activated clotting time test (ACT) of approximately 300 s, the first step will be the catheterization of the lowest renal artery, with the aim of leaving a guidewire as a marker for endograft placement. To facilitate fluoroscopic visualization, the branched endograft has proximal and distal markers, anterior and posterior markers, and a spatial orientation marker (tick marker). In addition, each side-branch has three markers on the proximal inner edge and two on the distal outer edge (Fig. 9.4).

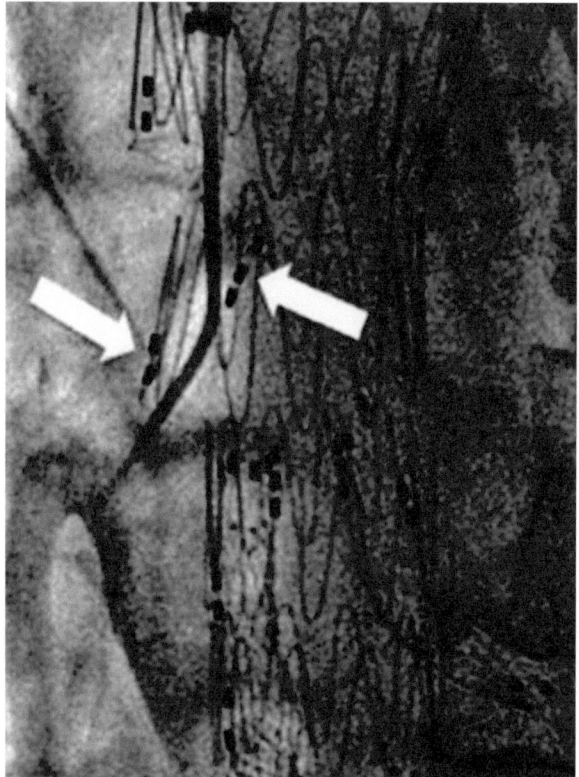

Fig. 9.4 Proximal and distal markers (arrows) identifying endoprosthesis branches

Assuming that any proximal thoracic components are to be placed as the first step of the procedure, the next step is to place the branch endoprosthesis through a femoral access. Before the complete deployment of the branched stent graft, it is necessary to ensure a proper overlap with the proximal thoracic component. It is also necessary to recognize the minimum distance between the renal artery marked by the guidewire left in place and the end of its side-branch (approximately 10 mm). The tick marker should also appear with the long side oriented to the left of the patient. As previously mentioned, the branched stent graft features a caliber reduction, after partial release, ensured by one or two reducing ties. This allows for manipulation (with extreme caution) of the endoprosthesis within the aorta to achieve the desired position based on the anatomy of the target arteries and thus facilitate catheterization. Once the endoprosthesis is completely unsheathed, after releasing of the reducing ties, the graft will be finally released in a definitive manner (Fig. 9.5). The procedure continues with the positioning and release of a distal bifurcated body and iliac extensions, with respect to patency of the internal iliac arteries. The stenting of the reno/visceral vessels, as already mentioned, can be performed from an arterial access of the upper limb or from below using a steerable introducer sheath. In both cases, it is preferable to use a coaxial system composed of a 12–14 Fr introducer in which a longer 8 Fr introducer will be inserted (Fig. 9.6). Once the catheterization of a target vessel has been performed through its side-branch, the standard hydrophilic guide wire used for selective catheterization is replaced with a stiffer Rosen-type guide wire (Cook Medical). At this point, a self or balloon-expandable covered stent can be introduced through the sheath and released in the correct position to bridge the space between the side-branch and the target vessel. Before the deployment of the bridging stent, care should be taken to ensure that the proximal end of the covered stent is at level of the proximal markers of the side-branch and there is an adequate distal landing within the target vessel, with respect to the patency of any division branches.

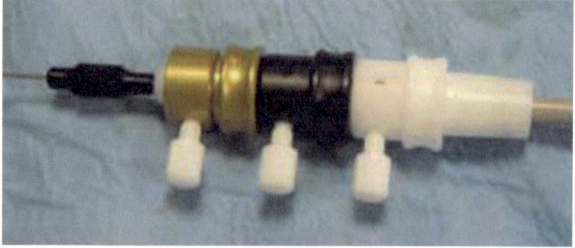

Fig. 9.5 Knobs connected to the releasing wires, used for complete release of the endoprosthesis

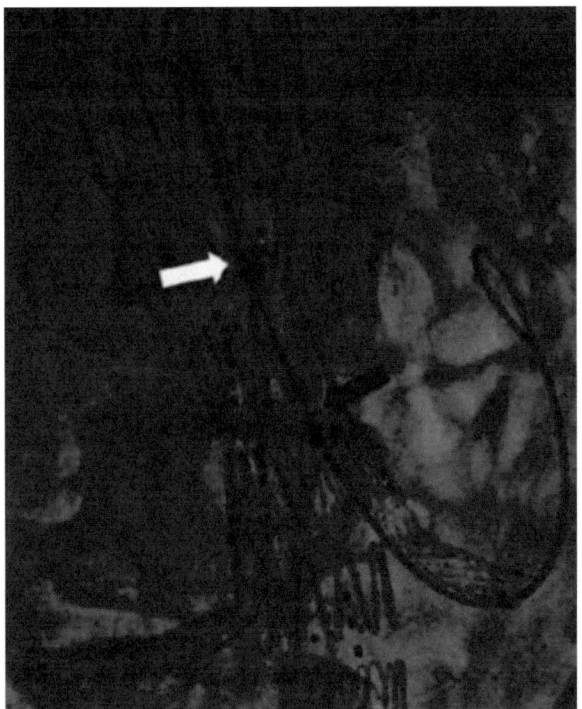

Fig. 9.6 Telescopic technique to catheterize a target vessel through its branch

Procedure: Fenestrated Endoprosthesis

Specific contraindications for current branch endoprosthesis designed with outer side-branches, such as a small internal aortic lumen typically observed in post-dissection TAAAs, may evoke the use of a custom-made fenestrated endoprosthesis. As mentioned, fenestrations must be precisely calibrated at the origin of the reno-visceral vessels. With the patient under general anesthesia in supine position, with the arms along the body and the upper limbs flected below the plane of the spine, in order to better visualize the origin of the target vessels also in lateral projection, the bilateral femoral approach is performed by surgical exposure or percutaneous technique. With an ACT test of approximately 300 s, after puncture of the femoral arteries, the first step will be the catheterization of the lowest renal artery, with the aim of leaving a guiding wire as a marker for endograft placement. All fenestrations present 4 markers positioned 90° apart. Assuming that any proximal thoracic components are to be placed as the first step of the procedure, the next step is to place the fenestrated endoprosthesis through a femoral access. Fenestrated grafts, as well, present a caliber reduction provided by one or two reducing ties. This allows manipulation of the endoprosthesis within the aorta to achieve the desired position based on the anatomy of the target arteries and thus facilitate their catheterization. In cases of pronounced tortuosity of the aorta, abnormal torsion of the fenestrated graft may occur, despite correct orientation during introduction. This can represent a critical moment in the procedure, which can be resolved with cautious and minimal adjustments during release. Once the endoprosthesis has been completely unsheathed, the fenestrated graft is catheterized through the distal end, from the contralateral femoral access, with a standard hydrophilic guidewire, then replaced with a stiffer Lunderquist-type guidewire (Cook Medical). An introducer sheath, generally 18–20 Fr, inserted on this guidewire, will be the working channel for catheterization of the target vessels through each fenestration. Small introducer sheaths (generally 6–7 Fr) will be inserted into this working channel through which the target vessels will be catheterized. The higher the number of target vessels catheterized before the complete release of the endoprosthesis, the safer and efficacious will be the procedure in terms of technical success related to stenting and patency of reno-visceral vessels. The standard hydrofilic guidewire used for catheterization of target vessels is replaced with a stiffer Rosen-type guidewire (Cook Medical). Then, the directional catheter is replaced by the tapered dilator of the introducer to facilitate its progression within the target vessel through the fenestration. The time required to catheterize target vessels through fenestrations remains a critical point of the procedure, especially for downward-facing arteries, which may require the use of an approach from above or the use of a steerable introducer sheath. To achieve a catheterization of target vessels from above, a preloaded catheter, designed at the time of customization and inserted into the delivery system through one or more fenestrations during device construction, may be useful. Where catheterization of a target vessel from above is not possible, progression of an introducer from below into a caudally directed artery can be extremely difficult. In these cases, catheterization of the target vessel may be performed using a steerable introducer sheath, if necessary. When all target vessels have been catheterized through each fenestration, the fenestrated stent graft can be fully and definitely deployed by removing the releasing wires that partially constrain and engage it in the delivery system. Before the placement of the bridging stents, it is necessary to ensure that the most proximal third of each balloon-expandable bridging stent protrudes approximately 8–10 mm into the lumen of the fenestrated endograft and that there is an adequate landing (at least 2 cm) within the target vessel. A proper protrusion of the covered stent is essential to obtain the so-called flaring that ensures its engagement with the fenestrated main body. The flaring can be obtained by using an angioplasty balloon (10–12 mm in diameter and 20 mm in length) inflated in the most proximal part (the one protruding inside the fenestrated endoprosthesis) of the balloon-expandable covered stent. The procedure is completed with the placement and release of a straight or bifurcated endoprosthesis and any iliac extensions, if needed.

Follow-Up

All patients undergoing advanced aortic repair with branched or fenestrated devices should be advised that the treatment they have received requires regular and ongoing follow-up to evaluate the performance of their endovascular implant. Patients should be informed about the importance of adhering to a specific follow-up program, both during the first year after surgery and at annual intervals thereafter. Patients should be informed that adequate and regular follow-up is a crucial part of the treatment they have received and is essential to ensure the safety and efficacy of the technique in the long run. The recommended imaging program includes a CT angiography scan before discharge (or alternatively a 1 month after the procedure), and at 6 and 12 months after surgery and annually thereafter (at least for the first 5 years). An X-ray of the abdomen can be a valid alternative for the identification of possible stent fractures or migration and/or disconnection phenomena. This schedule continues to be the minimum requirement for follow-up of patients and should be maintained even in the absence of symptoms. Patients with specific findings such as endoleaks, residual aneurysmal sac growth, and/or changes in the structure or position of endovascular components should be followed up at more frequent intervals. Annual follow-up imaging should include abdominal radiographs and CT examinations. If any deterioration of renal function precludes the use of contrast medium, abdominal radiographs, CT scans without contrast medium, and duplex ultrasound may be used. The combination of these methods can provide important information on any changes in residual aneurysm diameter, endoleak, patency of target vessels, progression of aneurysmal disease, and other morphological changes. Abdominal radiographs provide information on device integrity (separation between components, fractures, and migration). Ultrasonographic imaging can provide information on the maximum diameter of the residual aneurysmal sac, endoleak, and patency of the reno-visceral vessels; however, in the follow-up of advanced aortic procedures, ultrasonography may be a less accurate diagnostic method than CT angiography, and in case of doubtful findings it should always be complemented by a second-tier method.

Secondary Operations

Separation of endograft components and their migration may be factors responsible for aneurysm reperfusion. Type Ic and III endoleak, which is relatively rare with standard aortic endovascular procedures, can potentially become more frequent with increasing complexity and number of modular junctions. Secondary correction of these complications represents one of the most common causes of re-intervention after branched and fenestrated procedures. In a recent publication from the Cleveland Clinic, the authors analyzed a cohort of 650 patients undergoing endovascular treatment of complex aortic aneurysms with branched and fenestrated endografts. The mean follow-up in this cohort was 3 years, and during the maximum follow-up of 9 years, secondary procedures were required in 6% of cases for right renal artery, 5% for left renal artery, 0.6% for celiac trunk, and 4% for superior mesenteric artery. Death due to complications related to a target vessel occurred in three patients, all with problems inherent to superior mesenteric artery [18]. Complications related to target vessels may involve ischemic issues as well as reperfusion of the aneurysm. Type Ic or III endoleak complicating an advanced aortic procedure should in any case be considered a high flow endoleak and therefore always represents an indication for re-intervention. If it occurs lately (acute endoleak), the clinical presentation may be very similar to an aneurysm rupture. Both insufficient landing into the target vessels and disconnection of the bridging stents from the aortic endoprosthesis can be managed by percutaneous procedures, preferably under local anesthesia. In these cases, the aim of re-intervention is to realign the bridging stent along its entire length, from the proximal attachment zone to the target vessel, in order to reconnect the endovascular components and ensure patency of the target vessel and sealing the aneurysm again (Fig. 9.7).

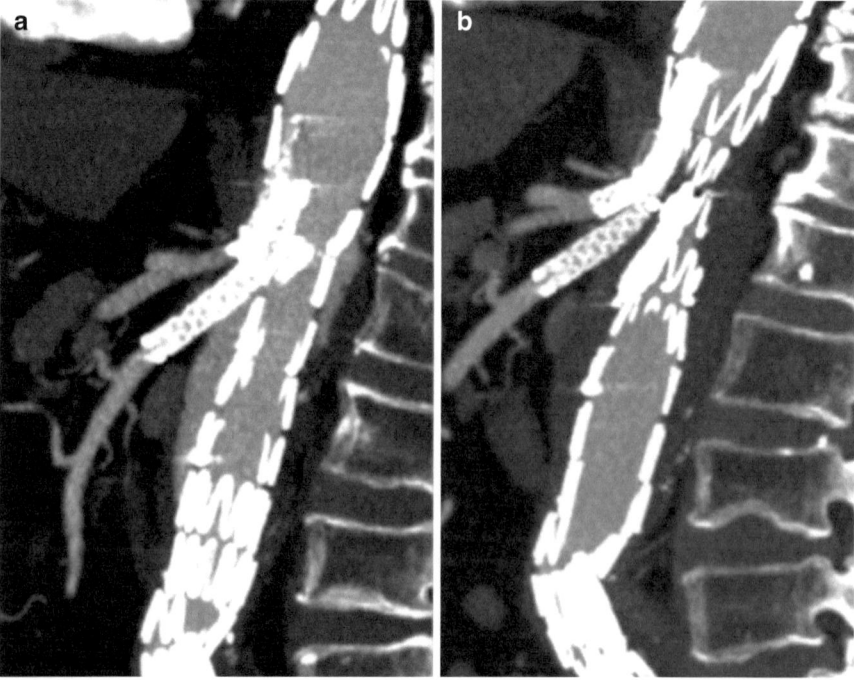

Fig. 9.7 Post-contrast CT multiplanar reconstructions with maximum intensity projection (MIP) before (**a**) and after (**b**) "relining" procedure on the celiac tripod, which aimed to disconnect the previous stent from the target vessel

References

1. Frederick JR, Woo YJ. Thoracoabdominal aortic aneurysm. Ann Cardiothorac Surg. 2012;1(3):277–85.
2. Crawford ES, Hess KR, Cohen ES, et al. Ruptured aneurysm of the descending thoracic and thoracoabdominal aorta. Analysis according to size and treatment. Ann Surg. 1991;213:417–25; discussion 425–6.
3. Heijmen RH, Deblier IG, Moll FL, et al. Endovascular stent-grafting for descending thoracic aortic aneurysms. Eur J Cardiothorac Surg. 2002;21:5–9.
4. Makaroun MS, Dillavou ED, Kee ST, et al. Endovascular treatment of thoracic aortic aneurysms: results of the phase II multicenter trial of the GORE TAG thoracic endoprosthesis. J Vasc Surg. 2005;41:1–9.
5. Ferrer C, Cao P, De Rango P, et al. A propensity-matched comparison for endovascular and open repair of thoracoabdominal aortic aneurysms. J Vasc Surg. 2016;63:1201–7.
6. Gallitto E, Faggioli G, Pini R, et al. Endovascular repair of thoraco-abdominal aortic aneurysms by fenestrated and branched endografts. Eur J Cardiothorac Surg. 2019;56(5):993–1000.
7. Greenberg RK, Clair D, Srivastava S, et al. Should patients with challenging anatomy be offered endovascular aneurysm repair? J Vasc Surg. 2003;38:990–6.
8. Ducasse E, Lepidi S, Brochier C, et al. The open chimney graft technique for juxtarenal aortic aneurysms. With discrepant renal arteries. Eur J Vasc Endovasc Surg. 2014;47(2):124–30.
9. Gallitto E, Gargiulo M, Freyrie A, et al. Off-the-shelf multibranched endograft for urgent endovascular repair of thoracoabdominal aortic aneurysms. J Vasc Surg. 2017;66(3):696–704.e5.
10. Chuter TA, Gordon RL, Reilly LM, et al. An endovascular system for thoracoabdominal aortic aneurysm repair. J Endovasc Ther. 2001;8:25–33.
11. Rolls AE, Jenkins M, Bicknell CD, et al. Experience with a novel custom-made fenestrated stentgraft in the repair of juxtarenal and type IV thoracoabdominal aneurysms. J Vasc Surg. 2014;59:615–22.
12. Greenberg R, Eagleton M, Mastracci T. Branched endografts for thoracoabdominal aneurysms. J Thorac Cardiovasc Surg. 2010;140(6 Suppl):S171–8.
13. Verzini F, Loschi D, De Rango P, et al. Current results of total endovascular repair of thoracoabdominal aortic aneurysms. J Cardiovasc Surg (Torino). 2014;55:9–19.
14. Verhoeven EL, Katsargyris A, Bekkema F, et al. Ten-year experience with endovascular repair of thoracoabdominal aortic aneurysms: results from consecutive166 patients. Eur J Vasc Endovasc Surg. 2015;49:524–31.
15. Conrad MF, Crawford RS, Davison JK, et al. Thoracoabdominal aneurysm repair: a 20-year perspective. Ann Thorac Surg. 2007;83:S856–61; discussion S890–2.
16. Shiga T, Wajima Z, Apfel CC, et al. Diagnostic accuracy of transesophageal echocardiography, helical computed tomography, and magnetic resonance imaging for suspected thoracic aortic dissection: systematic review and meta-analysis. Arch Intern Med. 2006;166:1350–6.
17. Yoshida S, Akiba H, Tamakawa M, et al. Thoracic involvement of type A aortic dissection and intramural hematoma: diagnostic accuracy—comparison of emergency helical CT and surgical findings. Radiology. 2003;228:430–5.
18. Mastracci TM, Greenberg RK, Eagleton MJ, et al. Durability of branches in branched and fenestrated endografts. J Vasc Surg. 2013;57:926–33.

Abdominal Aortic Aneurysm

10

Pier Giorgio Nardis, Simone Ciaglia, Bianca Rocco, Simone Zilahi de Gyurgyokai, Alessandro Cannavale, and Carlo Catalano

Introduction

Abdominal aortic aneurysms (AAAs) are classified according to their location and relationship to the renal arteries, as illustrated in Fig. 10.1.

- Infrarenal aneurysm: the sac is located below the origin of the renal arteries, with the possibility of identify a tract of healthy aorta (named as proximal neck).
- Iuxtarenal aneurysm: the aneurismatic sac is located just below the origin of the renal arteries.
- Pararenal aneurysm: the renal arteries are involved by the aortic dilatation.
- Suprarenal aneurysm: the extension of the aneurysmatic dilatation is above the renal arteries origin.

The treatment indications for AAAs are:

- Aneurysms with a diameter of 5 cm in male and 4.5 cm in female (due to the higher rupture rate in smaller aortic size that occur in women compared to men) [1, 2];
- Aneurysm growth rate more than 5 mm in 6 months or 10 mm in 1 year;
- Symptomatic aneurysms (distal embolization, rupture or impending rupture) [3, 4].

P. G. Nardis (✉) · S. Ciaglia · B. Rocco · S. Z. de Gyurgyokai · A. Cannavale · C. Catalano
Vascular and Interventional Radiology Unit, Department of Radiological, Oncological and Anathomo-Patological Science, Policlinico Umberto I, "Sapienza" University of Rome, Rome, Italy
e-mail: p.nardis@policlinicoumberto1.it; alessandro.cannavale@uniroma1.it; carlo.catalano@uniroma1.it

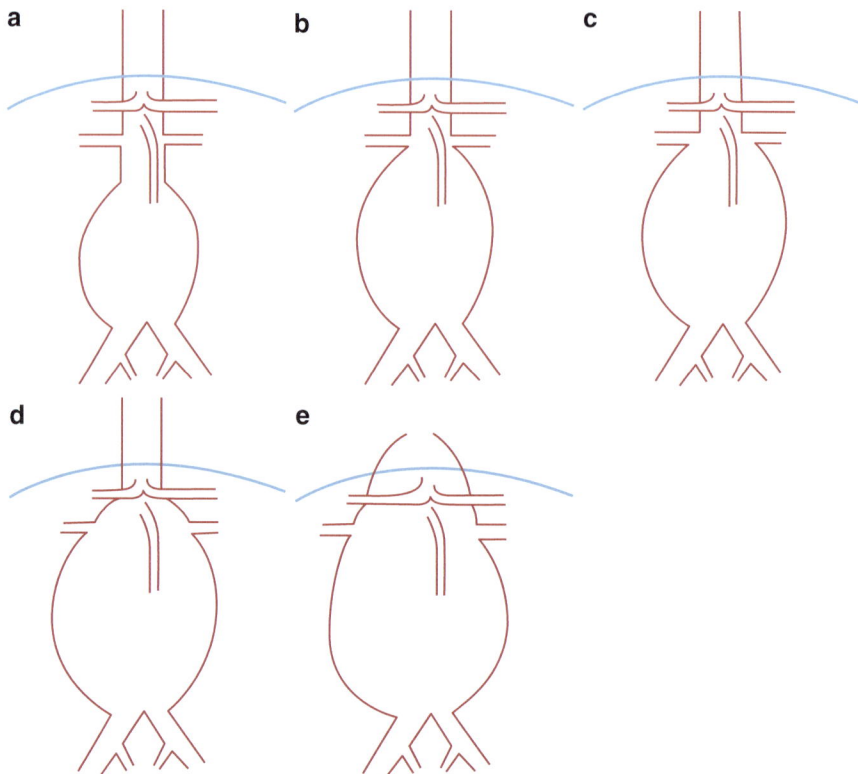

Fig. 10.1 Summary diagram of the classification of AAAs: (**a**) infrarenal aneurysm, (**b**) iuxtarenal aneurysm, (**c**) pararenal aneurysm, (**d**) suprarenal aneurysm, and (**e**) thoracoabdominal aneurysms

In the last two decades, abdominal endovascular aneurysm repair (EVAR) has become the first choice for AAA treatment; in the USA, approximately 80% of all AAAs are treated with EVAR [5].

Aortic endoprosthesis are covered self-expanding stent that exclude the aneurysm from blood flow. They consist of a self-expandable metal cage made in nitinol or cobalt chromium, coated by an impermeable layer of polytetrafluoroethylene (ePTFE).

Fig. 10.2 Example of an aortic endoprosthesis: (**a**) aortic main body, (**b**) iliac modules

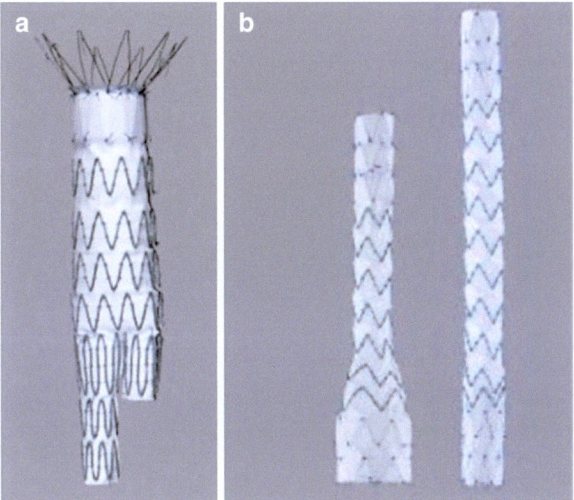

The definitive endoprosthesis implant results from assembling different components, with the most frequent configuration being an aortic stent, also named main body, placed into the aorta, and two iliac branches, consisting in two stents that connect the main body to the iliac arteries (Fig. 10.2).

Generally endoprosthesis are introduced into the aorta by transfemoral access (Fig. 10.3a, b). Once the desired position is reached, the main body of the endoprosthesis is released and it regains its normal conformation thanks to its shape memory (Fig. 10.3c); this allows the stent to adhere to the aortic wall.

Afterwards, iliac stents are released in order to connect the main body of the endoprosthesis to the iliac arteries, obtaining the complete exclusion of the aneurysm from the blood flow (Fig. 10.3d–f).

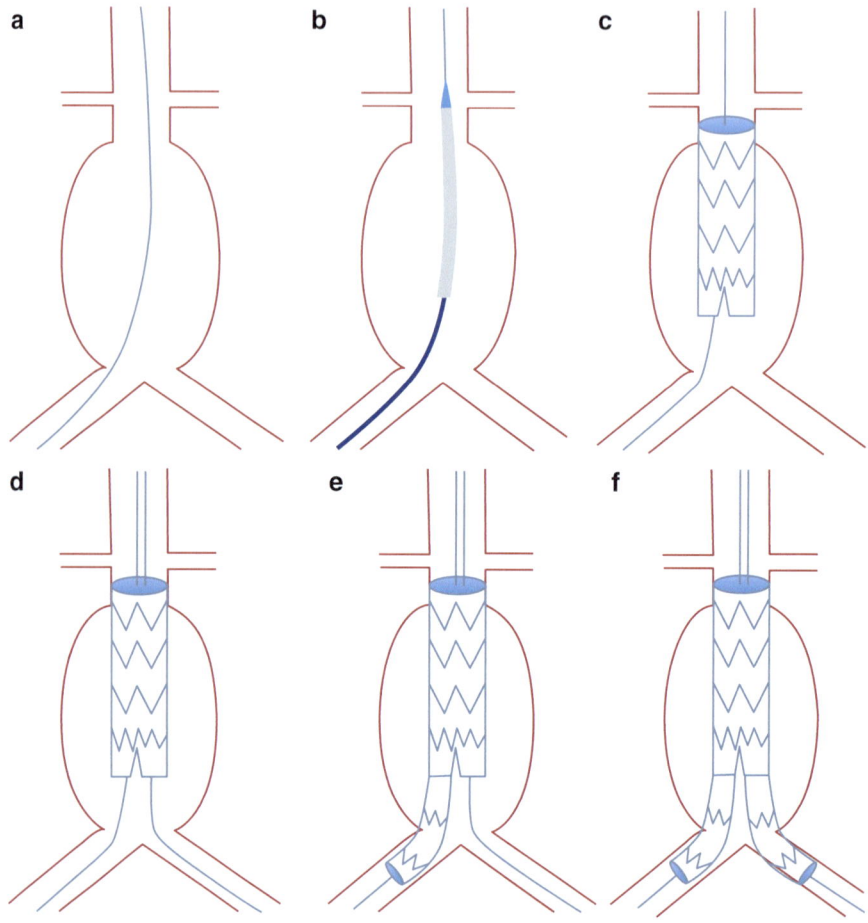

Fig. 10.3 Stages of placement and release of abdominal aortic endoprosthesis: from the transfemoral arterial access a guidewire (**a**) and then the main body of the aortic endoprosthesis are advanced into the aorta (**b**); the endoprosthesis is then released at the desired position (**c**). From the contralateral arterial access, the gate of the iliac module is gained (**d**), and both iliac components are placed (**e** and **f**), with an optimal overlap with the main body, with complete exclusion of the aortic aneurysm

CT Characteristics

Vascular Access: Common Femoral Arteries and Iliac Arteries

Femoral and iliac arteries represent the access to the arterial system, allowing to introduce guidewires, catheters, and sheaths for endoprosthesis placement; arteries's characteristics influence the type of endoprosthesis to be choose. Although superficial arteries such ad common femoral arteries can be evaluated by color Doppler ultrasound examination, CT angiography is mandatory for pre-planning assessment and should include information on femoral and iliac vessels. In addition, while in the past vascular accesses were surgically exposed, nowadays arterial percutaneous approach is the method of choice. For this reason, it is even more necessary to provide information about the characteristics of the arteries.

1. *Caliber*: The most common delivery systems have a caliber ranging from 4 mm to 6 mm, hence an adequate vessel diameter is required; the iliac arteries represent the distal landing zone of the iliac components of the stent graft therefore a correct sizing of the vessel is mandatory in order to obtain adequate sealing.
2. *Plaques or wall alterations, tortuosity*: the presence of parietal calcified plaque on common femoral arteries makes the artery stiffer and therefore the passage of the delivery systems may be difficult with increased risk for vascular lesions (dissections, ruptures) as well as may limit the use of the closure systems [6]; also the tortuosity of the vessels could make difficult the implantation and navigation.
3. *Previous surgery*: previous endarterectomy, bypass, vascular patching.

Proximal Neck

The proximal aortic neck is defined as the distance between the lowest renal artery and the proximal extremity of the aneurysm and its anatomy influences the type of the endoprosthesis (7). Proximal neck's characteristics that have to be considered for the adhesion of the endoprosthesis and proper exclusion of the aneurysm are listed below [6–8]:

1. *Length*: the measurement has to be taken on multiple planes, using MPR with the main axis along the proximal aortic neck, from the origin of the lowest renal artery to the aneurysmatic sac (Fig. 10.4a–b).
2. *Diameter*: The measurement should be made using appropriate multiplanar reconstruction, perpendicular to the main axis of the aneurysm neck (Fig. 10.4b–d). In cases of tapered neck, the maximum and the minimum size should be reported and the choice of endoprosthesis will be adapted on the basis of this range.
3. *Angle*: the angle of the neck is calculated by the intersection of two lines, respectively, parallel to the main aortic axis and the neck axis (Fig. 10.5); angles greater than 150° are generally favorable, whereas angles less than 120° can made EVAR difficult with high risk of endoleak.
4. *Vessel wall*: the presence of plaques, thrombus, circumferential irregularity, can affect the seal of the endoprosthesis. A vessel wall disease with a thickness >2 mm is considered significant; (50% of the circumference is considered severe, 50%–25% moderate, less than 25% mild [8].

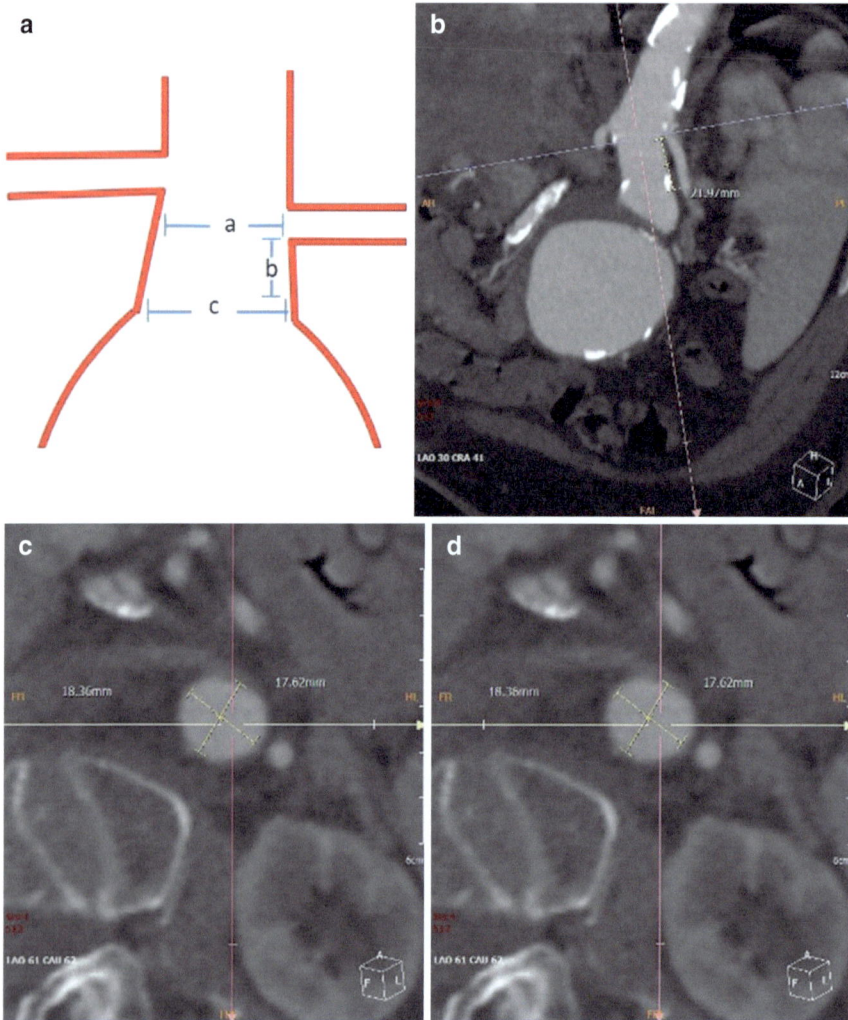

Fig. 10.4 Aortic aneurysm with markedly angulated collar. (**a**) Summary of neck measurements. (**b–d**) neck diameter measurement should be performed orienting the multiplanar reconstruction according to the main axis of the neck

Aorto-Iliac Anatomy

The following anatomical characteristics of the aorta and iliac arteries should be considered and described for the planning of EVAR.

1. *Aortic morphology*: aneurysms can be distinguished according to the shape (i.e., sacciform and fusiform).

Fig. 10.5 Angle of the proximal collar of the aneurysm

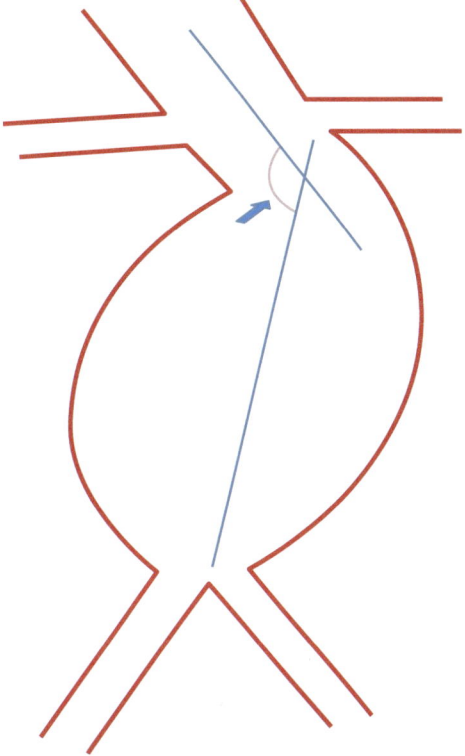

2. *Aortic length and iliac vessels*: the length of the aorta, measured from the origin of the lowest renal artery to the aortic bifurcation, and the length of the iliac arteries; these informations are mandatory for the sizing of the endoprosthesis.
3. *Aortic tortuosity*: the tortuosity of the aneurysm is evaluated using the aortic tortuosity index. This index is obtained by the ratio between a curved line drown in the center of the aorta from the lowest renal artery and the aortic bifurcation (Fig. 10.6 Line 1) and a straight line from the origin of the lowest renal artery and the aortic bifurcation (Line 2), in the coronal multiplanar reconstruction. Values greater than 1, 2 indicate a rather tortuous anatomy with difficulties for endoprosthesis positioning [6].
4. *Aortic arterial branches*: collateral branches arising from the AAA, mainly inferior mesenteric artery, lumbar arteries, accessory renal arteries should always be reported, since they are involved in type II endoleak development [9].
5. *Aortic bifurcation caliber*: the diameter of the aortic bifurcation must be evaluated to ensure proper expansion of the iliac limbs of endoprosthesis (at least 18–20 mm) [10].

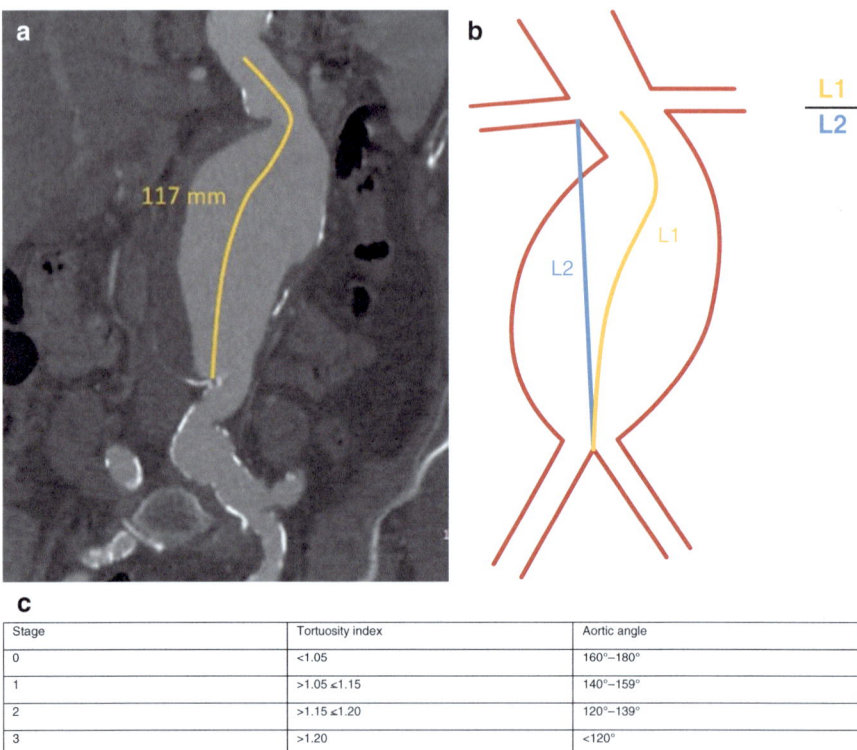

Fig. 10.6 (**a**) Curved Planar Reconstruction (CPR) for aortic length evaluation. (**b**) Summary diagram for evaluation of the tortuosity index. (**c**) Reference table

Type of Endoprosthesis

Different types of endoprosthesis are available in the market and the selection depends on aortic and neck morphology and wall characteristics.

Infrarenal and Iuxtarenal Aneurysms

There are different stent graft for the treatment of infrarenal aneurysms:

1. *Endoprosthesis with infrarenal fixation*: the stent graft is totally covered and therefore has to be positioned below the origin of renal arteries; it requires adequate proximal neck length (at least 15–20 mm) and a favorable anatomy in order to obtain a correct adhesion of the stent-graft to the aortic wall (Figs. 10.7a and 10.8).

10 Abdominal Aortic Aneurysm

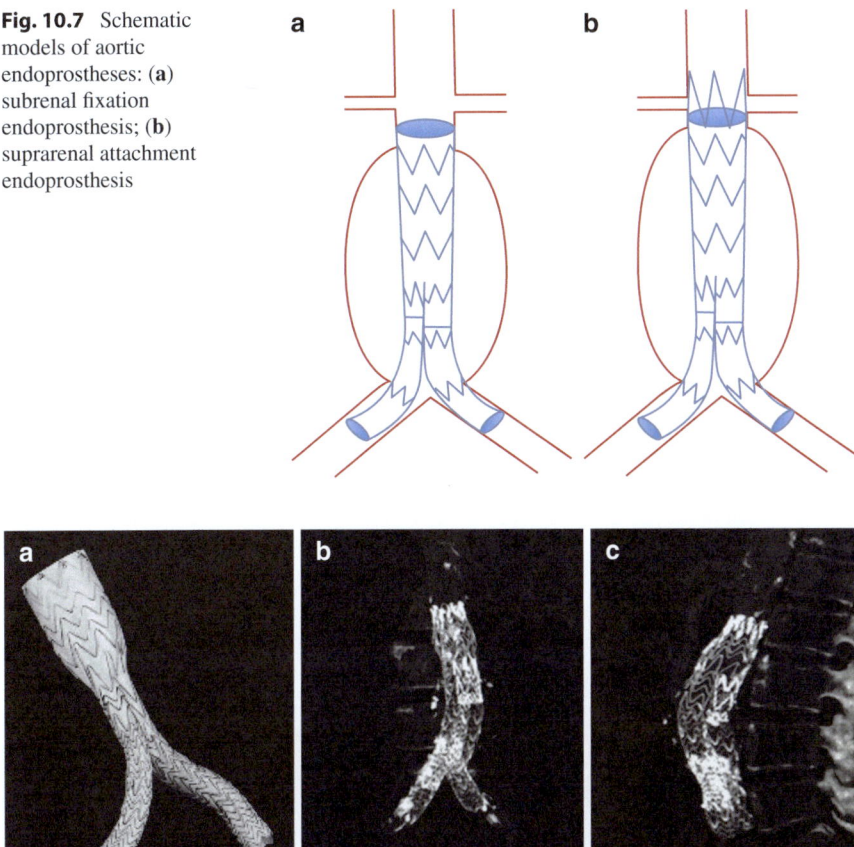

Fig. 10.7 Schematic models of aortic endoprostheses: (**a**) subrenal fixation endoprosthesis; (**b**) suprarenal attachment endoprosthesis

Fig. 10.8 Totally covered endoprosthesis with subrenal fixation (**a**); (**b**) MPR reconstruction—coronal projection; (**c**) MPR reconstruction—lateral projection

2. *Endoprosthesis with suprarenal fixation*: the proximal part of the stent graft presents an uncovered mesh and can be placed nearby and above the renal arteries, without compromising their patency; the majority of these type of endoprosthesis are equipped with hooks that allow the anchoring to the vessel wall (Figs. 10.7b and 10.9); this type of endoprosthesis is used in case of short and angulated proximal neck (<15–20 mm);
3. *Other endoprosthesis models*: some manufacturers have designed special stent graft that, due to their conformation and structure, aim to increase the adhesion to the neck (Fig. 10.10) and reduce the risk of endoleak (Fig. 10.11).

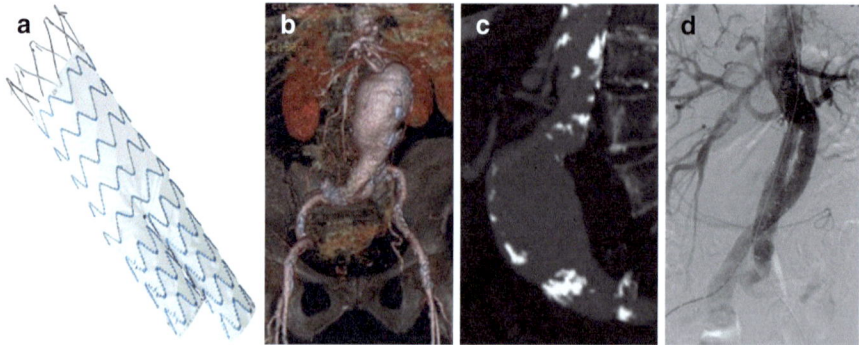

Fig. 10.9 Endoprosthesis with suprarenal fixation (**a**). Implantation performed on aortic aneurysm with markedly tortuous neck and anatomy; 3D and MPR reconstruction of a giant juxtarenal aneurysm with a short and tortuous neck (**b, c**); final angiogram after stent-graft deployment (**d**)

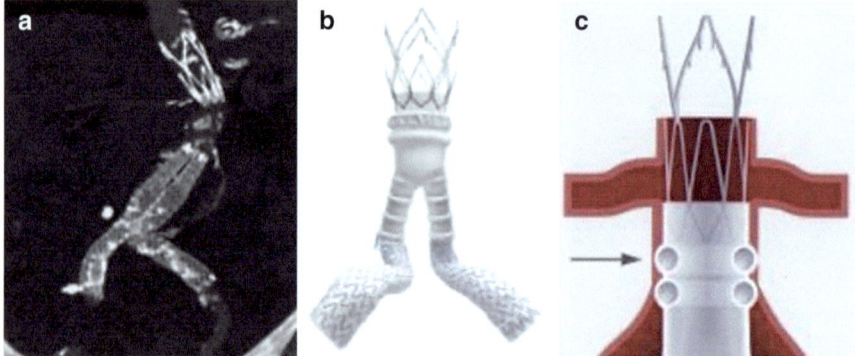

Fig. 10.10 (**a**) MPR reconstruction after stent-graft deployment; the polymer-filled ring structure promote adhesion of the endoprosthesis to the proximal neck wall (**b, c**)

Pararenal and Suprarenal Abdominal Aneurysms

In cases of pararenal or suprarenal aneurysms, standard endoprosthesis cannot be used; alternative techniques have to be considered to allow the aneurysm exclusion ensuring at the same time patency of the splanchnic vessels. Basically there are two techniques to treat this type of aneurysms: custom-made endoprostheses (in election), standard fenestrated aortic stent graft and endoprosthesis with chimney, periscope, octopus technique (in emergency).

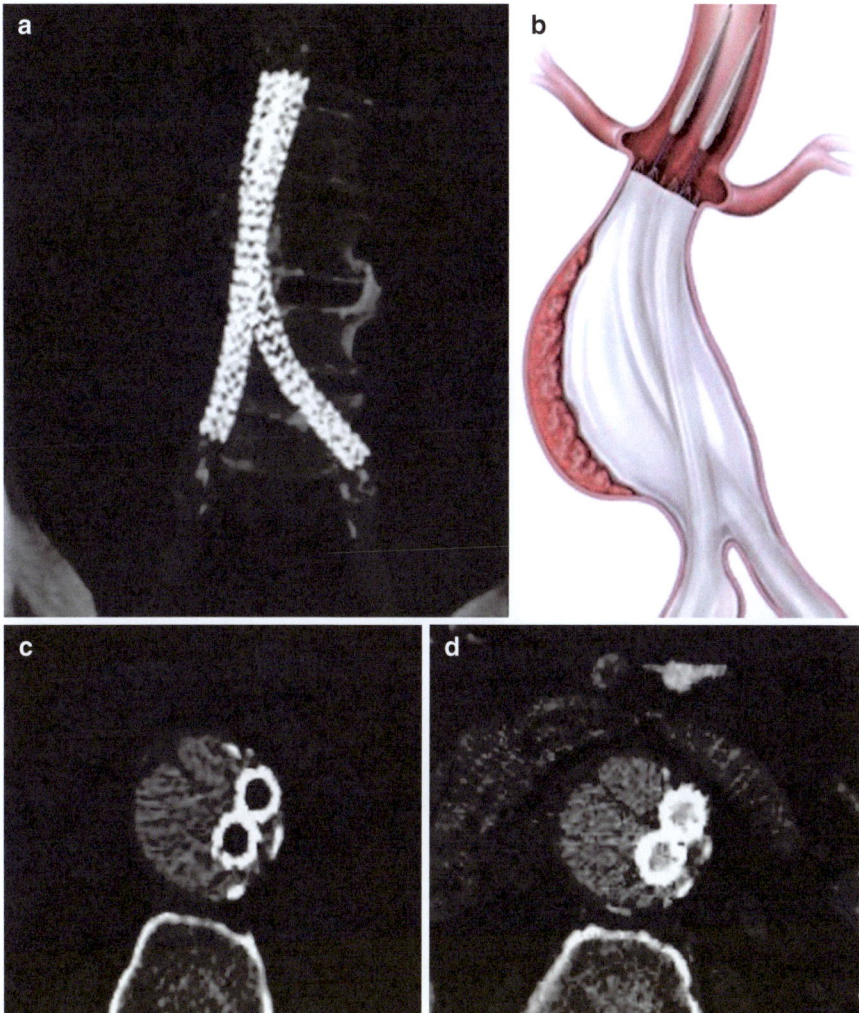

Fig. 10.11 (**a**, **b**) Endoprosthesis consisting of two covered stents each with a bag (endobag) that is filled with a stable polymer (polyethylene glycol) to occupy the space in the sac. (**c**) Basal CT scan; note the hyperdensity of the polymer filling the endobag. (**d**) CT scan after mdc

Custom-Made Endoprosthesis

These endoprosthesis are tailored to the patient's aortic anatomy. Specifically, holes, scallops, or small branches are created on the main structure of the endoprosthesis at the level of the origin of the splanchnic vessels, allowing them to be catheterized and stented. Introduced in 1990 [11], the custom-made stent graft permitted to wide indications for the treatment of aortic pathology. In the last years some companies developed standard fenestrated or branched aortic stent graft suitable for patients that

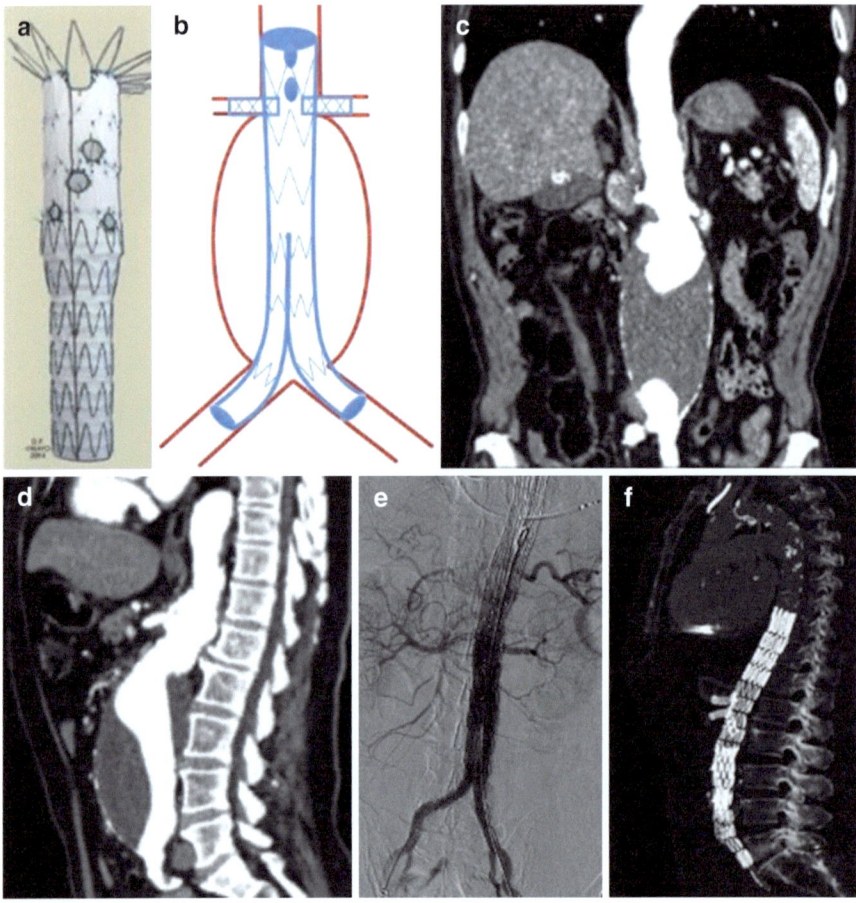

Fig. 10.12 (**a, b**) Model of fenestrated endoprosthesis with example implantation scheme. (**c–f**) Patient with pararenal aortic aneurysm treated with fenestrated endoprosthesis

present the origin of visceral arteries within a given range; these type of endoprosthesis are useful for elective aneurysm treatment but especially for emergency cases. Two different families of stent graft can be distinguished: fenestrated and branched.

1. *Fenestrated endoprostheses.* They can be made with scallops on the upper profile and holes at the origin of the splanchnic vessels (Fig. 10.12a, b). They are indicated in the treatment of pararenal and iuxtarenal aneurysms where the splancnic vessels are located in the neck.

    Once the holes of the endoprosthesis are properly aligned with the origin of the splanchnic vessels, covered stents are placed to connect the vessels to the main body (Fig. 10.12c–f).
2. *Branched endoprostheses.* These are custom-made endoprosthesis indicated for pararenal, suprarenal, and thoracoabdominal aneurysms, where the splanc-

10 Abdominal Aortic Aneurysm

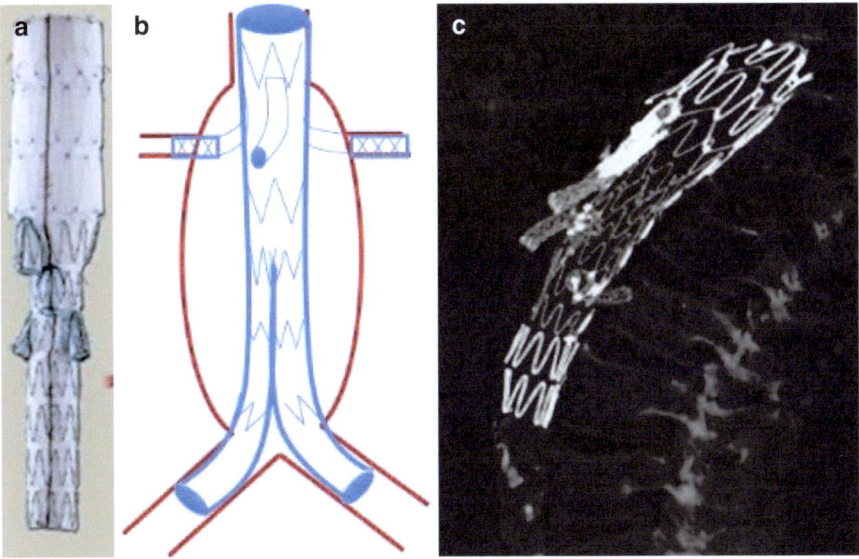

Fig. 10.13 Branched endoprosthesis for the treatment of suprarenal aneurysms: (**a**) model of branched endograft; (**b**) schematic example of a branched endograft; (**c**) MPR reconstruction of a CT scan performed 1 month after branched endoprosthesis deployment

nic vessel arise from the sac. In these cases, the origin of the splanchnic vessels are far from the main body of the endoprosthesis, requiring branches (Fig. 10.13a–c), that are subsequently connected to the splanchnic vessels by means of covered stents to achieve proper revascularization of the splanchnic vessels.

Chimney Endoprosthesis and Periscope Technique

Custom-made endoprosthesis fabrication takes several days, precluding their employment in emergency settings. Although there are standard branched endoprosthesis on the market based on the average of aortic anatomies, in most cases these are not applicable [12, 13]. Chimney technique was developed as salvage technique in case of incidental coverture of the renal artery by the stent graft and consists in covered stents placed parallel and external to the stent graft with the proximal end above (chimney technique) (Fig. 10.14a) or below (periscope technique) (Fig. 10.14b) the endoprosthesis end and into the splancnic vessel to revascularize. Currently, this technique is reserved in patients presenting juxtarenal, pararenal, or suprarenal aneurysms in emergency settings.

Unfortunately this technique presents high risk of complication especially Type I endoleak due to poor adhesion of the endoprosthesis to the aortic wall caused by the presence of stents located outside the main body (gutter endoleak) (Fig. 10.15). Moreover, in order to guarantee the patency of the covered stents to the splanchnic organs, antiplatelet therapy has to be performed thus influencing aneurysm sac thrombosis.

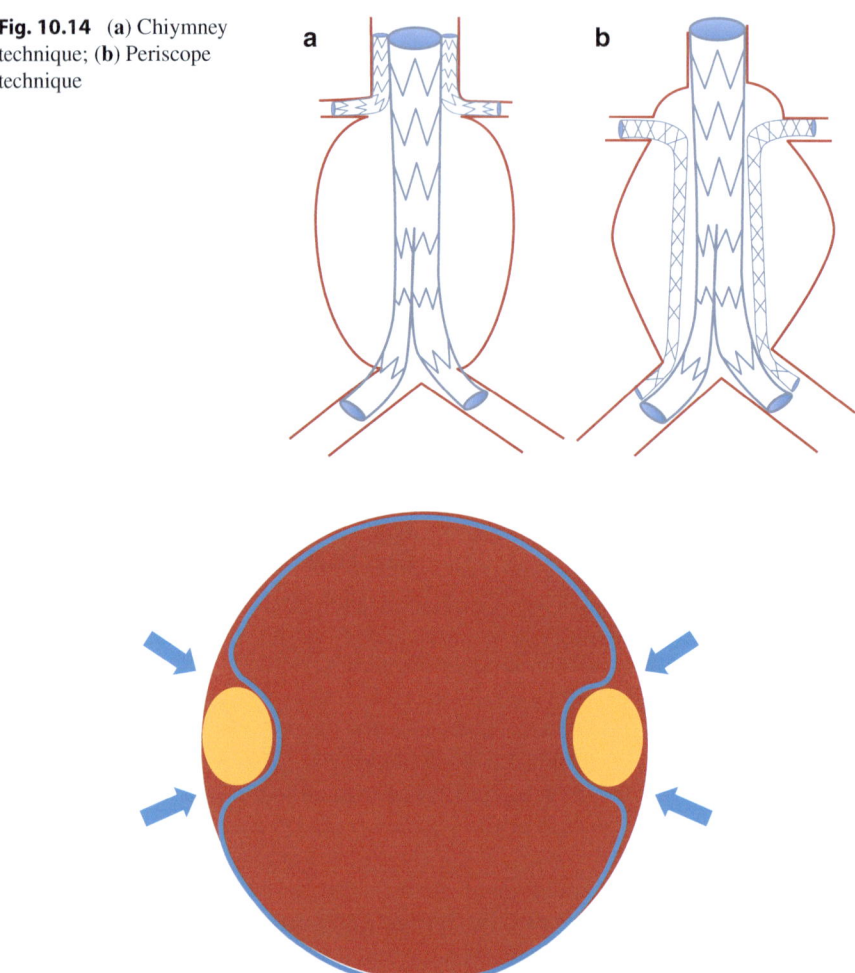

Fig. 10.14 (**a**) Chiymney technique; (**b**) Periscope technique

Fig. 10.15 Schematic cross-sectional image of an endoprosthesis implanted with chimney technique; note the areas of non-adhesion of the endoprosthesis to the aortic wall (arrows), resulting in potential endoleak

Further problems include the occlusion of the stents in the splanchnic vessels with consequent organ ischemia; for splanchnic vessels, longer stents are used with an increased risk of angulation and occlusion. For these reasons, the chimney technique is nowadays reserved only for emergency settings where standard techniques are not feasible (Fig. 10.16).

Iliac Arteries Aneurysm

Isolated iliac artery aneurysms are rare entities while more often aortic aneurysm may present with synchronous aneurysm of the iliac arteries; endovascular

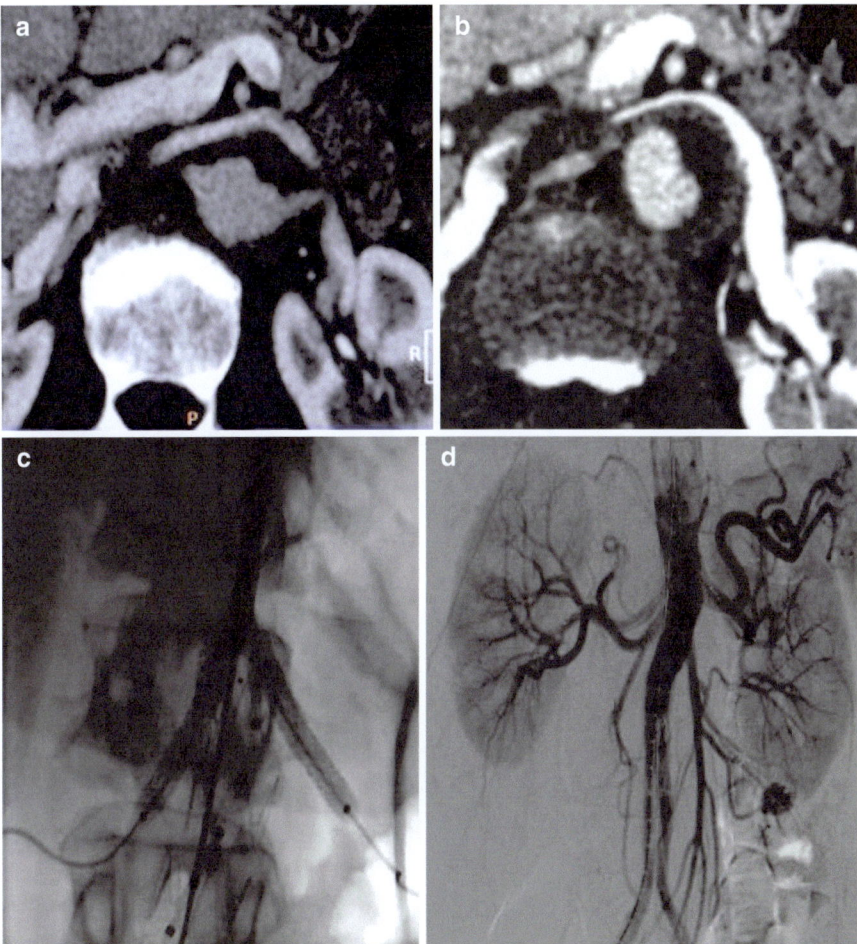

Fig. 10.16 (**a**, **b**) CT demonstrating a small pararenal aneurysm, with signs of impending rupture, in a young woman with abdominal pain. (**c**, **d**) Stent-graft with with chimney technique: stents are first placed in the renal arteries and then the endoprosthesis is deployed. Final angiography shows correct positioning of the stent graft, patency of both renal arteries and no signs of endoleak

treatment is the method of choice. If the aneurysm involves the intermediate tract of the common iliac artery, with favorable anatomy and suitable proximal and distal neck, a covered stent graft is generally enough to exclude the sac (Fig. 10.17). In some other cases, there is no sufficient neck for distal landing of the iliac endoprosthesis. Covering the origin of the hypogastric artery exposes to the risk of retrograde revascularization of the sac (type II endoleak) (Fig. 10.18a) [14]. There are different endovascular techniques for the treatment of iliac artery aneurysm involving the hypogastric origin [15].

Fig. 10.17 Schematic example of left aorto-iliac aneurysm treated by bifurcated aortic endoprosthesis extended to cover both aortic and left common iliac aneurysms

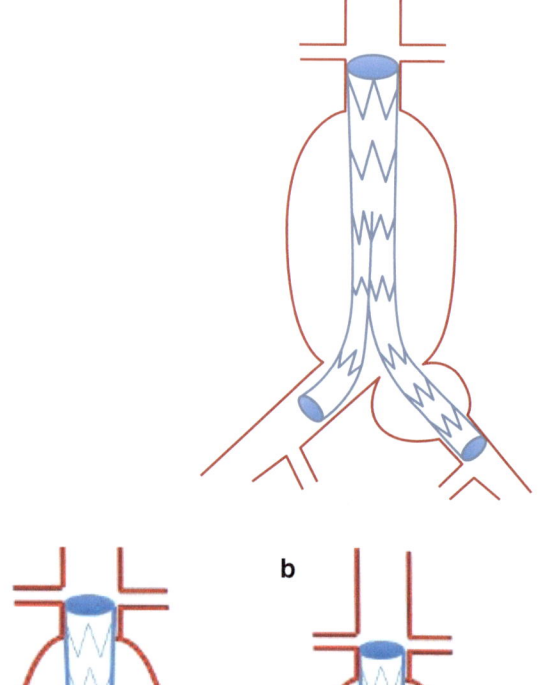

Fig. 10.18 Schematic example of left aorto-iliac aneurysm; the distal neck of the iliac aneurysm is insufficient: placement of the endoprosthesis distal to the origin of the hypogastric artery could cause retrograde revascularization of the aneurysmatic sac (type II endoleak) (**a**), so hypogastric artery embolization with metal coils is performed (**b**)

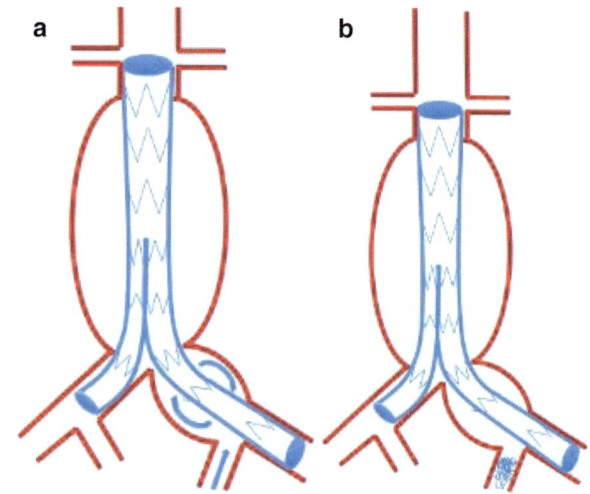

Internal Iliac Artery Embolization

Embolization of the hypogastric artery at the origin using metal coils or plugs is the most widespread technique; it is technically feasible with a low rate of major complications (Fig. 10.18b) [16, 17]. In fact, if the embolization is very close to the origin of hypogastric artery, a revascularization of the branches downstream is supplied by collaterals (gluteal, pudendal, bladder, and inferior hemorrhoidal arteries) with low risk of hypoperfusion disorders [18, 19]. This risk increases when both hypogastric arteries are embolized (i.e., in cases of bilateral iliac artery aneurysms) [20]. The most frequent complication observed after unilateral hypogastric embolization is gluteal claudication (26–41%); however, symptoms tend to regress with time due to the development of collateral circulation [21]. Guidelines recommend preservation of at least one hypogastric artery, if possible; when embolization of both hypogastric arteries is required, it is recommended to perform the treatment in two stages. More recently, branched endoprosthesis have been developed for preservation of the hypogastric axis in cases of iliac aneurysms.

Iliac Branch Endografts

As mentioned below, the current trend in the treatment of iliac aneurysms involving the origin of the hypogastric artery is preserving its patency, especially in young patients or in patients with bilateral iliac aneurysms (Fig. 10.19) [19]. Branched endoprosthesis present a prosthetic branch that can be released at the origin of the hypogastric artery; an additional covered stent is used to connect the branch of the main body of the endoprosthesis to the artery [22].

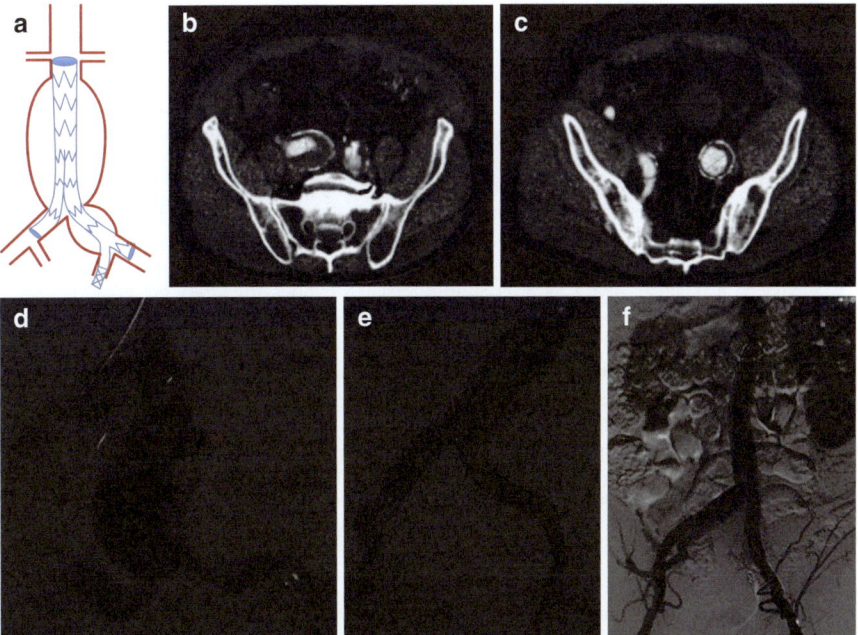

Fig. 10.19 (a) Schematic representation of a branched endoprosthesis for internal iliac artery. CT scan shows bilateral iliac aneurysm (b, c); placement of right iliac branch endoprosthesis (d, e); final angiogram after left internal iliac embolization with metal coils (f)

References

1. Antoniou GA, Georgiadis GS, Antoniou SA, et al. A meta-analysis of outcomes of endovascular abdominal aortic aneurysm repair in patients with hostile and friendly neck anatomy. J Vasc Surg. 2013;57(2):527–38.
2. Bryce Y, Rogoff P, Romanelli D, et al. Endovascular repair of abdominal aortic aneurysms: vascular anatomy, device selection, procedure, and procedure-specific complications. Radiographics. 2015;35(2):593–615.
3. Lederle FA, Powell JT, Greenhalgh RM. Repair of small abdominal aortic aneurysms. N Engl J Med. 2006;354:1537–8.
4. Powell JT, Brown LC, Forbes JF, et al. Final 12-year follow-up of surgery versus surveillance in the UK small aneurysm trial. Br J Surg. 2007;94:702–8.
5. Heikkinen M, Salenius JP, Auvinen O. Ruptured abdominal aortic aneurysm in a well-defined geographic area. J Vasc Surg. 2002;36(2):291.
6. Chaikof EL, Fillinger MF, Matsumura JS, et al. Identifying and grading factors that modify the outcome of endovascular aortic aneurysm repair. J Vasc Surg. 2002;35:1061–6.
7. McDonnell CO, Halak M, Bartlett A, Baker SR. Abdominal aortic aneurysm neck morphology: proposed classification system. Ir J Med Sci. 2006;175:4–8.
8. Tournoij E, Slisatkorn W, Prokop M, et al. Thrombus and calcium in aortic aneurysm necks: validation of a scoring system in a Dutch cohort study. Vasc Endovascular Surg. 2007;41:120–5.
9. Kim HO, Yim NY, Kim JK, et al. Endovascular aneurysm repair for abdominal aortic aneurysm: a comprehensive review. Korean J Radiol. 2019;20(8):1247–65.
10. Kouvelos GN, Antoniou G, Spanos K, et al. Endovascular aneurysm repair in patients with a wide proximal aortic neck: a systematic review and meta-analysis of comparative studies. J Cardiovasc Surg (Turin). 2019;60(2):167–74.
11. Resch T. Custom-made devices: current state of the art. EV Today. 2016;15(3):90–3.
12. Mehta M, Taggert J, Darling RC III, et al. Establishing a protocol for endovascular treatment of ruptured abdominal aortic aneurysms: outcomes of a prospective analysis. J Vasc Surg. 2006;44:1–8.
13. Ohki T, Veith FJ. Endovascular grafts and other image-guided catheter-based adjuncts to improve the treatment of ruptured aortoiliac aneurysms. Ann Surg. 2000;232:466–79.
14. Gelfand DV, White GH, Wilson SE. Clinical significance of type II endoleak after endovascular repair of abdominal aortic aneurysm. Ann Vasc Surg. 2006;20:69–74.
15. Bekdache K, Dietzek AM, Cha A, et al. Endovascular hypogastric artery preservation during endovascular aneurysm repair: a review of current techniques and devices. Ann Vasc Surg. 2015;29(2):367–76.
16. Rayt HS, Bown MJ, Lambert KV, et al. Buttock claudication and erectile dysfunction after internal iliac artery embolization in patients prior to endovascular aortic aneurysm repair. Cardiovasc Intervent Radiol. 2008;31:728–34.
17. Su WT, Stone DH, Lamparello PJ, Rockman CB. Gluteal compartment syndrome following elective unilateral internal iliac artery embolization before endovascular abdominal aortic aneurysm repair. J Vasc Surg. 2004;39:672–5.
18. Chaikof EL, Dalman RL, Eskandari MK, et al. The Society for Vascular Surgery practice guidelines on the care of patients with an abdominal aortic aneurysm. J Vasc Surg. 2018;67(1):2–77.e2.
19. Swerdlow NJ, Wu WW, Schermerhorn ML. Open and endovascular management of aortic aneurysms. Circ Res. 2019;124(4):647–61.

20. Bosanquet DC, Wilcox C, Whitehurst L, et al. Systematic review and meta-analysis of the effect of internal iliac artery exclusion for patients undergoing EVAR. Eur J Vasc Endovasc Surg. 2017;53(4):534–48.
21. Farivar BS, Abbasi MN, Dias AP, et al. Durability of iliac artery preservation associated with endovascular repair of infrarenal aortoiliac aneurysms. J Vasc Surg. 2017;66(4):1028–36.e18.
22. Malina M, Dirven M, Sonesson B, et al. Feasibility of a branched stent-graft in common iliac artery aneurysms. J Endovasc Ther. 2006;13(4):496–500.

Aortic Aneurysm in Emergency: Radiological Signs of Pre-Rupture and of Rupture

11

Nicolò Schicchi, Leonardo Teodoli, Pierleone Lucatelli, Paolo Esposto Pirani, Marco Fogante, Fatjon Cela, and Liliana Balardi

Clinical Scenario

In symptomatic cases, thoracic aortic aneurysm (TAA) may be suspected if there are clinical signs of compression of the periaortic structures, chest pain, aortic valve insufficiency or after the establishment of a complication such as dissection or rupture. Patients with tamponade TAA rupture usually show the onset of acute chest pain radiating into the retro-scapular region. In patients with symptomatic thoracoabdominal aneurysm, concomitant abdominal pain may also be present. Free TAA rupture usually leads rapidly to internal bleeding such as hemothorax and hemopericardium. Acute respiratory insufficiency may be the result of a free aortic rupture in the left hemithorax. Rarely, erosion into mediastinal structures may result in aorto-bronchial fistula with hemoptysis or aorto-esophageal fistula with hematemesis [1, 2]. The location of the rupture is very important because it determines the prognosis and the preoperative management. The closer the location of the aneurysm to the aortic valve, the greater the risk of death. Less than 50% of all patients with rupture arrive at the hospital alive; mortality can be as high as 54% at 6 h and 76% at 24 h after the initial event [3].

The classic presentation of a ruptured abdominal aortic aneurysm (AAA) includes abdominal pain, hypotension, and pulsatile abdominal mass; however, these symptoms may be present in less than 50% of cases [4]. Patients with tamponade AAA rupture may present with abdominal or back pain. In the presence of a free AAA rupture of an AAA, massive hemorrhage involving the perirenal or pararenal spaces, as well as free effusion into the peritoneal space, allows accurate diagnosis even with ultrasound. CT-angiography (CTA), however, is the imaging method of choice in the evaluation of patients with suspected free or tamponade rupture. CTA is considered the gold standard examination, with a sensitivity of 100% and specificity of 98–99% [5].

CT Acquisition Protocol and Reporting Notes

CTA evaluation of aortic aneurysm involves a triphasic angiographic study, with a pre-contrastographic phase, an arterial phase, and a venous phase.

Pre-contrastographic acquisition provides important information regarding the presence of wall calcifications and intramural hematoma and simultaneously allows an assessment of the lung parenchyma, mediastinum, abdominal organs, and retroperitoneal space [6].

The arterial phase involves the acquisition of thoracoabdominal thin-layer images (<1 mm thick) with intravenous administration of contrast material at high flows (1.26-gI/s) with the use of bolus test or bolus tracking (method to be preferred especially in critical patients).

The use of ECG gating, which should be reserved exclusively for patients in whom an ascending aortic problem is suspected, reduces pulsatility artifacts, allowing the correct assessment of ascending aortic diameters and allowing precise measurements of aortic diameters necessary for prognostic and therapeutic purposes [7].

The venous phase performed 60–120 s after contrast material administration allows assessment of any contrast extravasation indicating low flow intimal lesions, organ perfusion defects, and aortic wall rupture.

Imaging should also include the iliac and femoral arteries to provide information necessary for endovascular treatment planfication.

In some cases, preoperative imaging may reveal the possible presence of iliac or hypogastric aneurysms, occlusive disease in the iliac or renal arteries, the presence of congenital vascular anomalies, or aneurysmal involvement of splanchnic aortic branches.

CT Signs of Impending Aortic Aneurysm Wall Rupture (Pre-Rupture): Unstable Aortic Aneurysm

CT signs suggestive of impending rupture of an aortic aneurysm (pre-rupture) can be modest and easily underestimated. When these signs are present, the aortic aneurysm is defined unstable (UAA). Signs of imminent rupture of an aortic aneurysm are:

- *growth of the aneurysmal sac greater than 10 mm per year* compared to the previous CT scan (Figs. 11.1 and 11.2);
- *hyperdense crescent sign (high attenuation)* that can be referred to intramural hematoma, visible in the pre-contrastographic phase as a sickle-shaped area of hyperattenuation in the context of the aortic wall or parietal thrombus (Fig. 11.3);

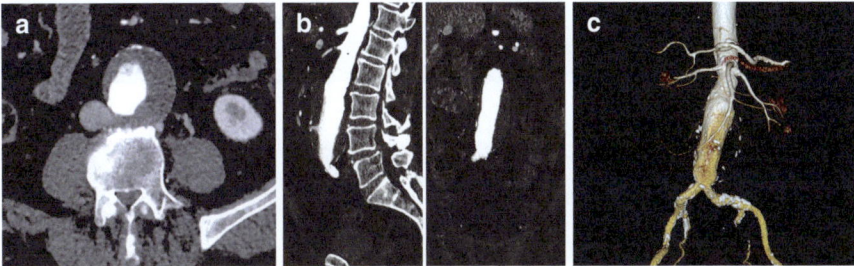

Fig. 11.1 Large AAA with endoluminal thrombosis. Post-contrast axial (**a**), multiplanar (**b**), reconstructions, 3D volume rendering (**c**)

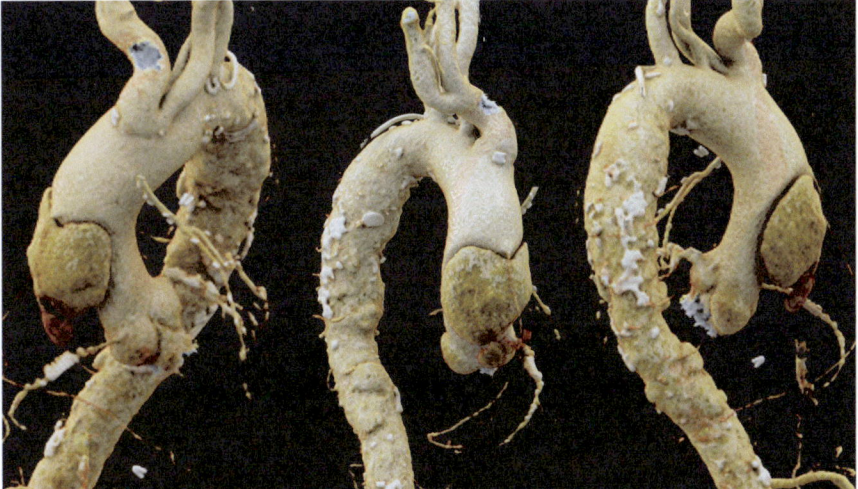

Fig. 11.2 Wall tear in the aneurysmal tract of the ascending thoracic aorta (3D Volume Rendering reconstructions)

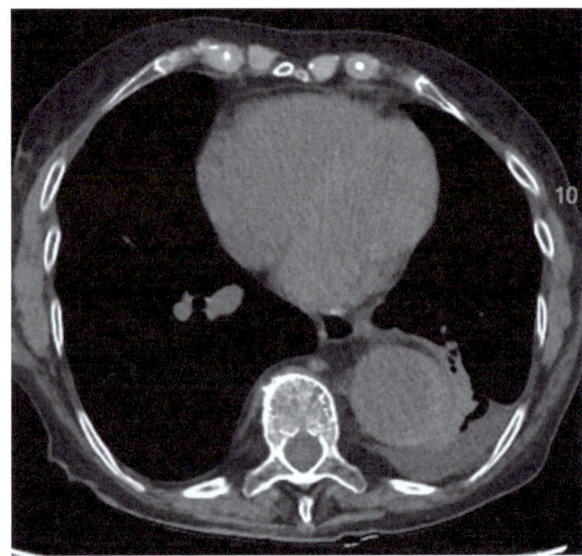

Fig. 11.3 Hyperdense crescent sign Intramural hematoma presents as a focal thickening, concentric or with half-moon morphology, of the aortic wall that appears hyperdense in the pre-contrast phase

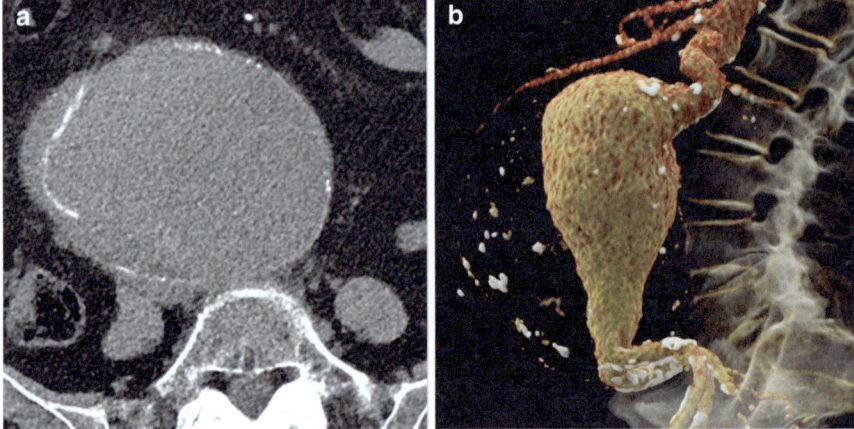

Fig. 11.4 Focal discontinuity of intimal calcification. In this case, it appears that the intimal calcification is moving away from the circumference drawn by the contour of the aneurysm. (**a**) Pre-contrast axial image; (**b**) 3D volume rendering

- *focal discontinuity of the intimal calcification or tangential calcification sign* with the intimal calcifications are distanced from the circumference delineated by the aneurysm (Fig. 11.4);
- *sign of "aortic draping"* with the posterior aortic wall is poorly defined and tightly adhered to the dorsal spine (Fig. 11.5);
- *increased ratio of lumen to parietal thrombus thickness* or the presence of an eccentric aortic lumen;

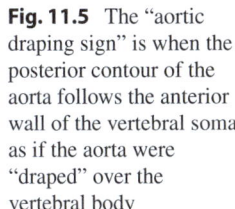

Fig. 11.5 The "aortic draping sign" is when the posterior contour of the aorta follows the anterior wall of the vertebral soma as if the aorta were "draped" over the vertebral body

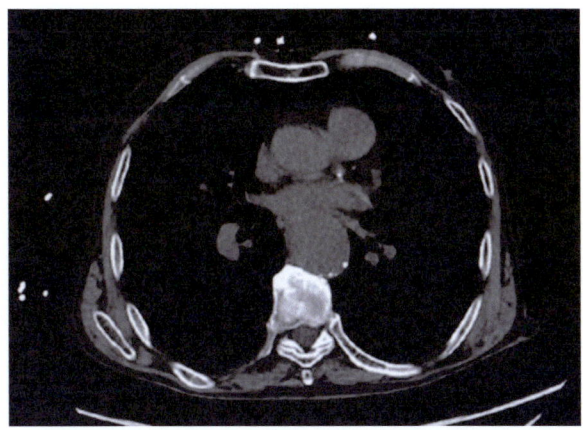

– *infection of the aneurysm sac*: infected (mycotic) aneurysms are rare, accounting for only 0.7–2.6% of aortic aneurysms. The rupture rate of infected aneurysms is 53–75%. Dissemination to the aneurysm sac occurs hematogenously in the context of septicemia, usually caused by endocarditis. A difference of atherosclerotic-based aneurysms, the most frequent site of mycotic aneurysms is thoracic or suprarenal abdominal. On CT examination, irregular contours, air bubbles, and signs of inflammation of the periaortic adipose tissue with possible abscess formation may be observed. Rapid change in size or shape of the aneurysm should raise suspicions about the possible presence of infection, indeed the rate of expansion of mycotic aneurysms is faster than that of atherosclerotic aneurysms.

CT Signs of Aortic Aneurysm Wall Rupture

Pre-contrastographic scan allows the recognition of the hematic hyperdensity of the collection, while post-contrastographic arterial scanning provides information about the size of the aneurysmal sac, the relationships with splanchnic and renal vessels and the site of rupture recognizable as a discontinuity of the wall associated with active overflow of contrast material into the para-aortic space. Primary signs of rupture of AAA are:

– *extravasation of contrast material*: the presence of hemomediastinum, hemopericardium, and hemothorax are clear signs of TAA rupture (Figs. 11.6 and 11.7), instead in AAA rupture, hematic collections may form retroperitoneally (Fig. 11.8) and extend to the perirenal space, pararenal space bilaterally and psoas muscles and intraperitoneal extension is less frequent and occurs late,
– *periaortic stranding*: diffuse hyperdensity of peripheral adipose tissue adjacent to the aneurysm;
– *retroperitoneal hematoma*: hyperdense fluid collection in the retroperitoneal space near the aneurysmal dilatation is one of the most important pathognomonic signs of AAA rupture;
– *aorto-enteric* fistula with the duodenum (most commonly III and IV portions) and symptoms such as abdominal pain, hematemesis, and melena.

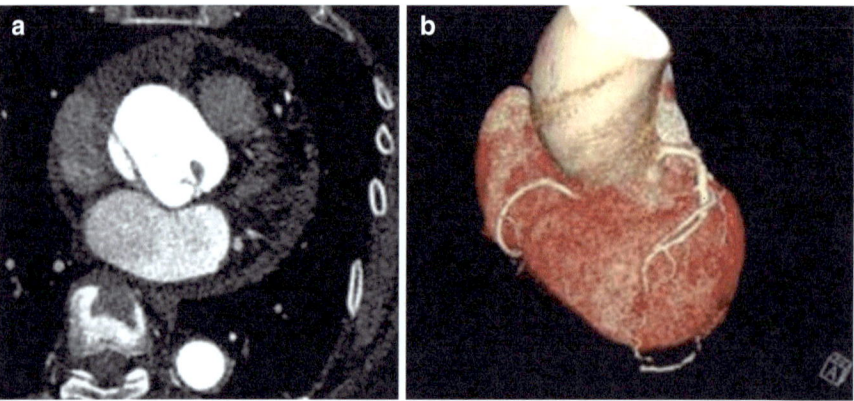

Fig. 11.6 Dissection of the ascending aorta (Stanford A) with intimal flap floating into the aortic lumen. Circumferential hemopericardium is associated. (**a**) Post-contrast axial CT image; (**b**) 3D volume rendering

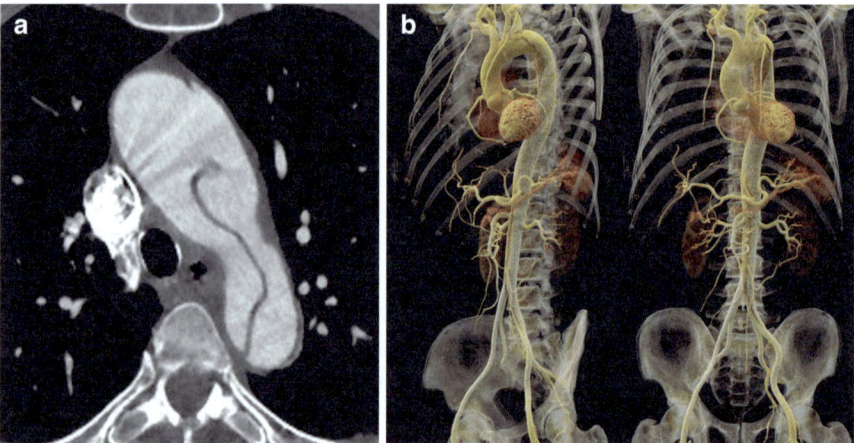

Fig. 11.7 Dissection of the thoracic aorta (Stanford B) with intimal tear in the aortic arch. (**a**) Contrast axial image; (**b**) 3D volume rendering

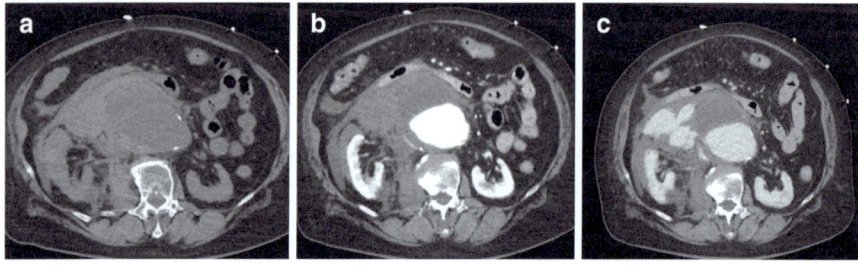

Fig. 11.8 Axial scan of massive abdominal aortic rupture with associated hematoma in retroperitoneum in pre-contrastographic phase (**a**), arterial phase (**b**), and venous phase (**c**)

References

1. Davis PM, Gloviczki P, Cherry KJ Jr, et al. Aorto-caval and ilio-iliac arteriovenous fistulae. Am J Surg. 1998;76(2):115–8.
2. Lemos DW, Raffetto JD, Moore TC, Menzoian JO. Primary aortoduodenal fistula: a case report and review of the literature. J Vasc Surg. 2003;37(3):686–9.
3. Johansson G, Markström U, Swedenborg J. Ruptured thoracic aortic aneurysms: a study of incidence and mortality rates. J Vasc Surg. 1995;21(6):985–8.
4. Aggarwal S, Qamar A, Sharma V, Sharma A. Abdominal aortic aneurysm: a comprehensive review. Exp Clin Cardiol. 2011;16(1):11–5.
5. Biancari F, Paone R, Venermo M, et al. Diagnostic accuracy of computed tomography in patients with suspected abdominal aortic aneurysm rupture. Eur J Vasc Endovasc Surg. 2013;45(3):227–30.
6. Boules TN, Compton CN, Stanziale SF, et al. Can computed tomography scan findings predict "impending" aneurysm rupture? Vasc Endovascular Surg. 2006;40(1):41–7.
7. Zubair MM, de Beaufort HWL, Belvroy VM, et al. Impact of cardiac cycle on thoracic aortic geometry-morphometric analysis of ECG gated computed tomography. Ann Vasc Surg. 2020;65:174–82.

Reporting Checklist: Endovascular Pre-Treatment

12

Bianca Rocco, Simone Ciaglia, Pierleone Lucatelli, Carlo Catalano, and Pier Giorgio Nardis

1. **Descending thoracic aortic aneurysm, intramural hematoma, atherosclerotic penetrating ulcer, rupture (descriptive elements)** (Fig. 12.1)
   (a) Morphology (fusiform, sac-like).
   (b) Location (proximal, middle, distal).
   (c) Extension (possible proximity and involvement of left subclavian).
   (d) Aneurysm diameter.
   (e) Angle.
   (f) Signs of rupture/impending rupture (yes/no).
   (g) Proximal neck (length, diameter, atherosclerotic plaques, angle).
   (h) Distal neck (length, diameter, atherosclerotic plaques, angle).
   (i) Presence of vessels originating from the sac (intercostal, spinal).
   (j) Presence of associated abdominal aortic aneurysms.
   (k) Iliac and femoral vessels (caliber, tortuosity, atherosclerotic plaques, previous surgery).
2. **Thoracic aortic dissection** (Fig. 12.2),
   (a) Type:
      - A: (valvular plane, ascending thoracic aorta, aortic arch).
        – Epiaortic vessels dissection (yes/no).
      - B: (descending thoracic aorta).
   (b) Extension.
   (c) Total aortic diameter.
   (d) True lumen diameter.

B. Rocco (✉) · S. Ciaglia · P. Lucatelli · C. Catalano · P. G. Nardis
Vascular and Interventional Radiology Unit, Department of Radiological, Oncological and Anathomo-Patological Science, Policlinico Umberto I, "Sapienza" University of Rome, Rome, Italy
e-mail: carlo.catalano@uniroma1.it; p.nardis@policlinicoumberto1.it

© The Author(s), under exclusive license to Springer Nature Switzerland AG 2024
I. Carbone et al. (eds.), *Imaging of the Aorta*,
https://doi.org/10.1007/978-3-031-52527-8_12

Fig. 12.1 Summary diagram of measurements to be provided for endovascular treatment of a thoracic aortic aneurysm: (**a**) proximal neck diameter; (**b**) proximal neck length; (**c**) distal neck diameter; (**d**) presence of vessels emerging from the aorta (neck and sac)

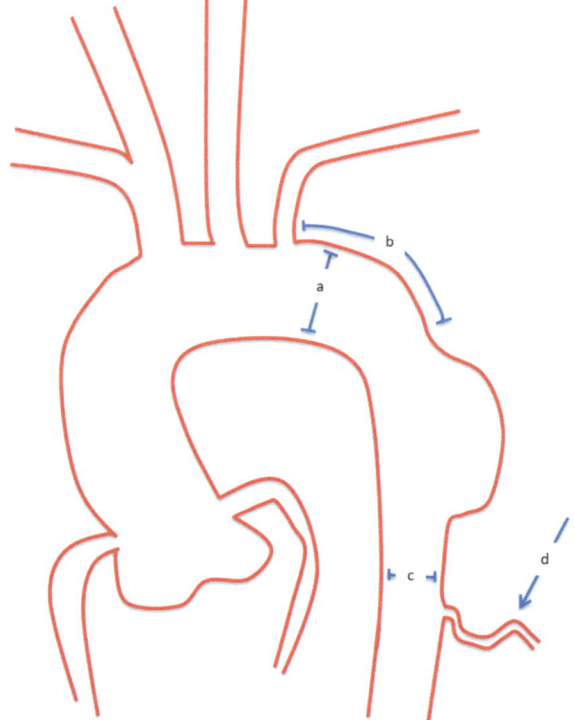

- (e) Signs of rupture/impending rupture.
- (f) Major intimal tear (location).
- (g) Visceral vessel involvement (possible organ ischemia),
- (h) Proximal neck (length, diameter, atherosclerotic plaques, angle).
- (i) Iliac and femoral vessels (caliber, tortuosity, atherosclerotic plaques, previous surgery).

3. **Abdominal aortic aneurysm** (Fig. 12.3),
    - (a) Morphology (fusiform, sac-like).
    - (b) Location (proximal, middle, distal).
    - (c) Extension.
        - Suprarenal.
        - Pararenal.
        - Iuxtarenal.
        - Infrarenal.

Fig. 12.2 Summary diagram of the information to be provided in case of aortic dissection. In addition to the informations provided in the previous diagram (Fig. 12.1), the presence and position of the dissecting intimal tears should be reported

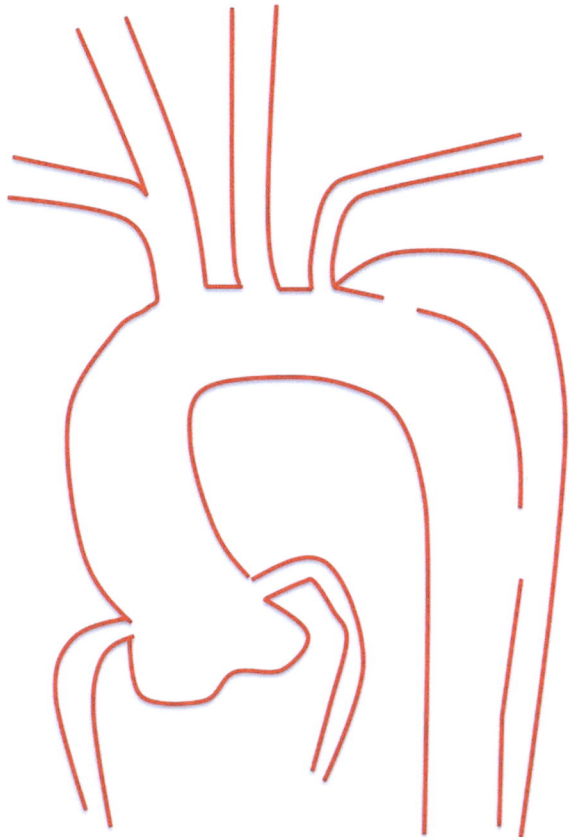

- (d) Aneurysm diameter.
- (e) Angle.
- (f) Signs of rupture/impending rupture (yes/no).
- (g) Proximal neck (length, diameter, atherosclerotic plaques, angle).
- (h) Distal neck (length, diameter, atherosclerotic plaques, angle).
- (i) Presence of vessels originating from the sac (accessory renal arteries, lumbar arteries, inferior mesenteric artery).
- (j) Presence of associated aneurysms (iliac aneurysms, hypogastric aneurysms).
- (k) Iliac and femoral vessels (caliber, tortuosity, atherosclerotic plaques, previous surgery).

Fig. 12.3 Summary diagram of measurements to be provided for endovascular treatment of an abdominal aortic aneurysm: (**a**) proximal neck diameter; (**b**) proximal neck length; (**c**) aorta length; (**d**) common iliac arteries length; (**e**) common iliac arteries caliber; (**f**) aortic Carrefour diameter; (**g**) femoral arteries diameter. The presence of visceral vessels arising from the sac or neck should also be noted

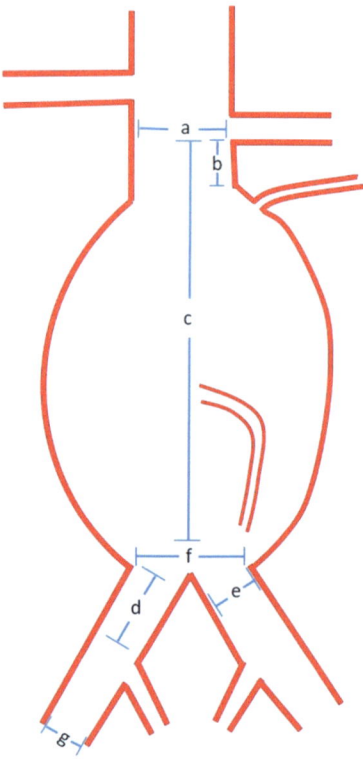

Part IV
Aortic Aneurysms: Follow-Up

Follow-Up After Endovascular Aneurysm Repair

Valentina Chiara Romano

Endovascular aneurysm repair (EVAR) is associated with a low incidence of periprocedural complications and mortality compared to open surgical repair (OSR). In the long term, however, this is counterbalanced by a relatively high incidence of secondary ruptures (2.1% vs. 0%), re-interventions (22.1% vs. 17.8%), and re-hospitalizations (21.4% vs. 17.8%), as well as higher mortality. Although more recent studies suggest a continuous decline in mortality after EVAR, a regular surveillance of the patients following endovascular treatment of aortic aneurysms is of vital importance [1].

The aim of aortic aneurysm repair—either by endovascular or surgical technique–is to contain arterial blood pressure and reduce aortic wall stress by channeling the blood flow into a graft, thus excluding the aneurysmal sac from the systemic circulation. The resulting thrombotic transformation with subsequent hypotrophy of the aneurysmal sac (within months/years) results in a progressive reduction of its diameter. In case of an endoleak, on the contrary, the blood flow persists within the aneurysmal sac which continues to be directly or indirectly exposed to systemic pressure. The eventual enlargement of the aneurysm is bound to an increasing danger of secondary rupture.

The objective of follow-up-imaging after EVAR is to allow the detection of medium- and long-term complications that may result in a secondary rupture of the aneurysm (high mortality event) and to allow planning of a secondary treatment or re-intervention.

While the early complications after endovascular repair are rather symptomatic, most late complications are due to the effect of hemodynamic stress on the endograft over the years and are asymptomatic and insidious.

V. Chiara Romano (✉)
Department of Radiology, Charité Universitaetsmedizin Berlin, Berlin, Germany

© The Author(s), under exclusive license to Springer Nature Switzerland AG 2024
I. Carbone et al. (eds.), *Imaging of the Aorta*,
https://doi.org/10.1007/978-3-031-52527-8_13

Imaging surveillance involves regular and lifelong follow-ups starting soon after the procedure. Patients undergoing EVAR are typically affected by complex pathologies, adequate imaging needs therefore to be efficient even in presence of associated chronic vascular alterations, such as atherosclerosis and calcification, stenosis, occlusion, and/or dissection.

For all these reasons, the role of the radiologist in terms of correct image interpretation, detection of relevant pathologies and well as structured and efficient reporting is crucial.

This chapter schematically focuses on the timing and imaging modalities for follow-up after endovascular aortic repair with the aim of sharpening up the vision of the reporter, with a particular focus on the detection of endoleaks, these being the most frequent complication after EVAR, often along with therapeutic consequences.

Examination Protocol

CT angiography is considered the gold standard for post-treatment surveillance of aortic aneurysms as it is effective in detecting migration, kinking, structural defects of the stent graft, endoleaks, infections, and aneurysm growth [2]. The standard surveillance protocol includes three phases: pre-contrast, arterial, and delayed [3].

Pre-contrast images serve to differentiate hyperdense calcifications from endoleaks that might appear in the following contrast enhanced phases. The late phase is decisive in detecting low-flow endoleaks that might otherwise remain occult in the earlier arterial phase. Angio-CT has a higher sensitivity in detecting endoleaks than angiography. The latter, however, allows dynamic visualization of the flow, accurate classification of the endoleak, and consequently the choice of treatment options (re-intervention vs. surveillance).

The maximum diameter of the aneurysmal sac should be accurately compared with that of the previous examinations. The use of a standardized measurement protocol helps to lower interobserver variability. The measurement tool should be used in the perpendicular plane to the axis of the aneurysm, ideally on "curved" MPRs (multiplanar reformatted images), the measurement being performed from the outer boundary of the aneurysm wall (adventitia-to-adventitia) [4]. In tortuous vessels and in the absence of MPRs, measuring the maximum diameter in the axial plane may be inaccurate. Nevertheless, if measurements are taken in a comparable way to previous follow-ups, i.e., using anatomical landmarks, changes in size can be identified with acceptable accuracy.

Cumulative radiation exposure, contrast media induced nephropathy, and cost are the risks or disadvantages to be taken into consideration in the use of CT angiography. The frequency of follow-up varies among different institutions and traditionally includes a baseline follow-up 1 month after EVAR, followed by surveillance intervals ranging from 6 to 12 months. In asymptomatic patients with aneurysms

<5 cm, or in those with a diameter reduction >5 mm during the first year after treatment, surveillance intervals may tend to be lengthened or CT angiography may be partially replaced by MRI or ultrasound.

Other Modalities

Ultrasound (duplex) can be technically challenging in obese patients, as well as in those with extensive arterial wall calcifications, but it can accurately reveal the diameter of the aneurysmal sac and allow precise visualization of proximal and distal anchoring sites in many cases [5]. The use of contrast enhanced ultrasound (CEUS) increases the sensitivity of plain ultrasound surveillance [6] and allows the classification of endoleaks by dynamically visualizing the flow direction in the aneurysm [7, 8].

Angio-MR can detect lumen patency, prosthesis placement, and residual flow in the aneurysm. Stents not made of nitinol but of stainless steel and cobalt-chromium-nickel alloy are ferromagnetic and may cause significant artifacts. Several studies suggest that angio-MR is more sensitive than angio-CT in detecting endoleaks [9]. In particular, in cases of suspected endotension (in which the aneurysm increases in size without an appreciable endoleak on imaging), angio-RM should be considered to identificate occult type II endoleaks in other modalities and avoid misclassification and wrong therapeutic choice. Non-enhanced MRI sequences provide an efficacious alternative to CT angiography in patients with renal insufficiency.

Radiographs in anteroposterior and lateral projection are useful for a comprehensive assessment of the position and integrity of the prosthesis. Complications such as stent graft migration, fractures, or kinking can be detected to supplement follow-up with MRI or ultrasound [10]. However, radiographs do not provide an assessment of the size of the aneurysmal sac and are not useful as a stand-alone screening modality.

Reporting the Post-EVAR Follow-Ups

The first and essential reporting step is the assessment of the maximum diameter of the aneurysm during the follow-ups. To do this, the instruments described above should be used, aiming to carefully repeat the measurements between the baseline examination and the current examination at an identical anatomical position. The detection of a shrinkage of the aneurysm makes the presence of an endoleak very unlikely. If the diameter of the aneurysm is unchanged or increasing, this strongly indicates the presence of an endoleak (Fig. 13.1).

Type I endoleak is caused by insufficient anchoring or "sealing" of the stent graft in its proximal (type Ia) or distal (type Ib) position, with consecutive blood flow outside the graft but within the aneurysmal sac and exposure of the latter to systemic arterial pressure. Angio-CT suggests the presence of a type I endoleak when a contrast media leak appears within the aneurysmal sac near the proximal or distal

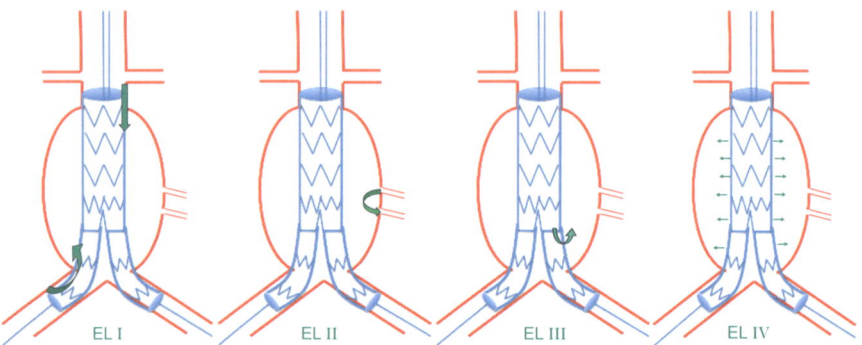

Fig. 13.1 Classification of endoleaks

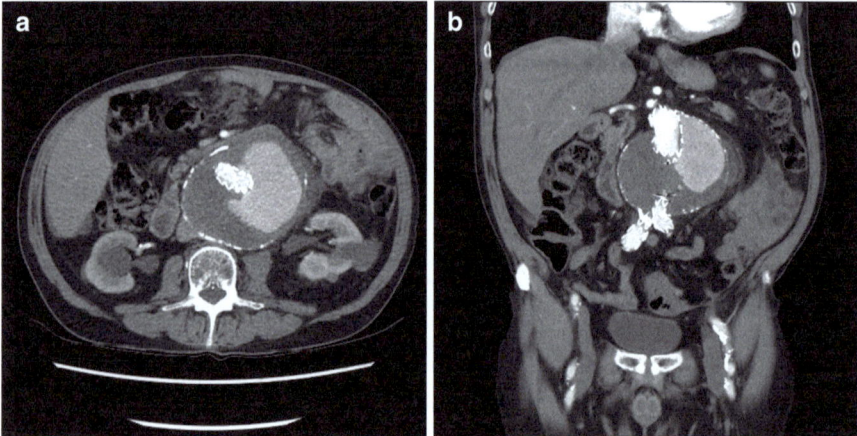

Fig. 13.2 Type I endoleak (**a**) and contained secondary abdominal aortic aneurysm rupture (**b**)

anchoring sites (Fig. 13.2). Typical risk factors for the occurrence of endoleaks of this type are an extended, angled, funnel-shaped, or calcified aneurysmal neck. In cases of type I endoleaks, early intervention is necessary to reduce the risk of secondary rupture. Treatment typically consists of reshaping the anchoring site by angioplasty, stenting, or endograft extensions. If the aneurysmal neck has expanded, placement of a fenestrated graft or chimney grafts may be an alternative to surgical conversion.

In type II endoleaks (25% of post-EVAR complications), the persistent flow within the aneurysm is supplied by at least two visceral branches ("entry" and "re-entry") of the aneurysm following flow reversal: typically, the inferior mesenteric artery (IMA) and/or the lumbar arteries. Some studies suggest that a large-caliber IMA is associated with a higher incidence of type II endoleak. Coil-embolization of the IMA prior to EVAR may consequently reduce its incidence. Up to 40% of type II endoleaks resolve spontaneously and immediate intervention is not always required (Fig. 13.3). Late type II endoleaks appear more than 1 year after aneurysm

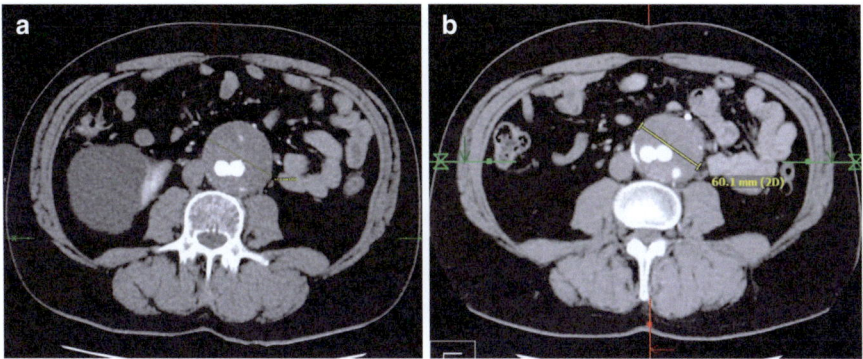

Fig. 13.3 Type II endoleak before (**a**) and after (**b**) coil-embolization of IMA. Three months after the procedure, a small endoleak persists while the diameter of the aneurysmal sac shows a decrease from 6.5 cm to 6.0 cm. No further intervention is necessary

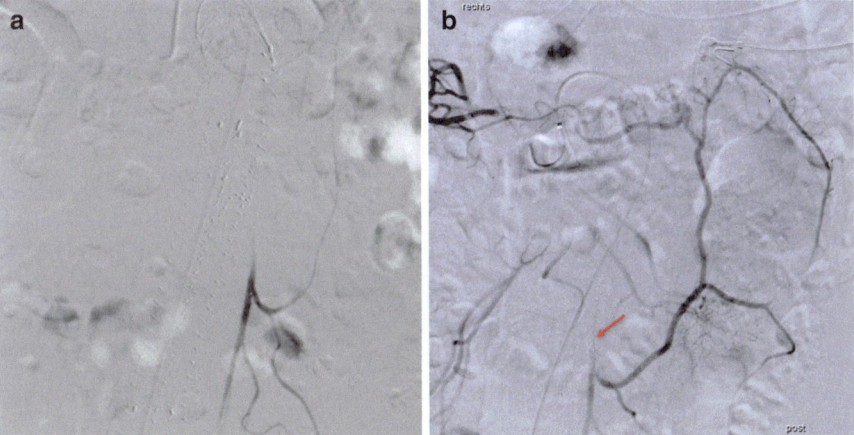

Fig. 13.4 (**a/b**) Endovascular coil-embolization of the IMA via arc of Riolan in a patient with type II endoleak associated with aneurysmal sac enlargement

treatment and are often associated with increased aneurysm size [11]. Endovascular treatment consists of embolization either by means of trans-arterial approach or direct CT-guided trans-lumbar puncture (Figs. 13.4 and 13.5).

In type III endoleak, blood flows directly into the aneurysm sac either because of a disconnection of the aortic module from the iliac module of the stent graft or because of a lesion of the prosthetic tissue. Angio-CT reveals a contrast media collection mostly adjacent to the endograft (and not in the periphery of the aneurysmal sac, as this is the case in type II endoleaks). Arterial pulsation and/or narrowing of the aneurysm may cause secondary distortion or migration of the stent graft and result in a secondary type III endoleak. Re-intervention is always necessary because of the rapid pressure buildup in the aneurysmal sac and the high risk of secondary rupture. Endovascular repair consists in the placement of a stent graft extension to

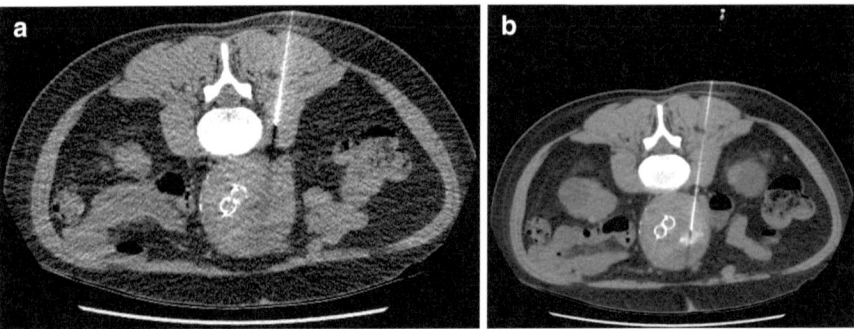

Fig. 13.5 (**a/b**) CT-guided percutaneous transluminal embolization of a type II endoleak associated with aneurysmal sac enlargement

Table 13.1 Endoleaks and treatment options

DIRECT ENDOLEAKS: re-intervention (always!) needed
Type I: Endovascular remodeling/extension with stent or stent graft
Type III: Endovascular sealing with stent graft/stent-in-stent to cover the breach
INDIRECT ENDOLEAKS: Primary follow-up, re-intervention in case of aneurysmal enlargement
Type II: Percutaneous translumbar embolization (CT-guided) or endovascular embolization (angiography)
Type IV/V: Surgical conversion (OSR)

reconnect the components or in the placement of a stent graft (stent-in-stent) to cover the breach.

In type IV endoleak, blood leaks from the stent graft because of the porosity of the prosthetic tissue. Along with the introduction of newer generation prostheses, this type of endoleak has become rare. Type V endoleak occurs when the aneurysm sac continues to increase in volume without an apparent cause (endotension).

The direct or indirect exposure of the aneurysmal sac to flow and thus to systemic arterial pressure determines whether re-intervention is mandatory or not. For this reason, endoleaks are further classified into "direct" or "indirect," the latter generally having a benign course (Table 13.1).

References

1. Li B, Khan S, Salata K, et al. A systematic review and meta-analysis of the long-term outcomes of endovascular versus open repair of abdominal aortic aneurysm. J Vasc Surg. 2019;70(3):954–969.e30.
2. van der Vliet JA, Kool LJ, van Hoek F. Simplifying post-EVAR surveillance. Eur J Vasc Endovasc Surg. 2011;42(2):193–4.

3. Rozenblit AM, Patlas M, Rosenbaum AT, et al. Detection of endoleaks after endovascular repair of abdominal aortic aneurysm: value of unenhanced and delayed helical CT acquisitions. Radiology. 2003;227(2):426–33.
4. Cayne NS, Veith FJ, Lipsitz EC, et al. Variability of maximal aortic aneurysm diameter measurements on CT scan: significance and methods to minimize. J Vasc Surg. 2004;39(4):811–5.
5. Back MR. Surveillance after endovascular abdominal aortic aneurysm repair. Perspect Vasc Surg Endovasc Ther. 2007;19:395–400.
6. Mirza TA, Karthikesalingam A, Jackson D, et al. Duplex ultrasound and contrast-enhanced ultrasound versus computed tomography for the detection of endoleak after EVAR: systematic review and bivariate meta-analysis. Eur J Vasc Endovasc Surg. 2010;39:418–28.
7. Iezzi R, Cotroneo AR, Basilico R, et al. Endoleaks after endovascular repair of abdominal aortic aneurysm: value of CEUS. Abdom Imaging. 2010;35:106–14.
8. Millen A, Canavati R, Harrison G, et al. Defining a role for contrast-enhanced ultrasound in endovascular aneurysm repair surveillance. J Vasc Surg. 2013;58:18–23.
9. Habets J, Zandvoort HJ, Reitsma JB, et al. Magnetic resonance imaging is more sensitive than computed tomography angiography for the detection of endoleaks after endovascular abdominal aortic aneurysm repair: a systematic review. Eur J Endovasc Surg. 2013;45:340–50.
10. Harrison GJ, Oshin OA, Vallabhaneni SR, et al. Surveillance after EVAR based on duplex ultrasound and abdominal radiography. Eur J Vasc Endovasc Surg. 2011;42:187–92.
11. Nolz R, Tuefelsbauer H, Asenbaum U, et al. Type II endoleak after endovascular repair of abdominal aortic aneurysms: fate of the aneurysm sac and neck changes during long-term follow-up. J Endovasc Ther. 2012;19:193–9.

Follow-Up of Untreated Aneurysm

14

Angelo Iannarelli and Giovanni Trillò

Conservative Management and Follow-Up of Uncomplicated Abdominal Aortic Aneurysm (AAA)

The choice of the most appropriate instrumental evaluation interval is relative to the caliber of the abdominal aorta at the time of diagnosis. The term ectasia/dilatation of the abdominal aorta is used when the vessel caliber reaches a maximum size between 2.5 and 2.9 cm.

An antero-posterior (DAP) or transverse (DT) diameter of the abdominal aorta between 3.0 and 5.5 cm is defined as a small aneurysm. The most appropriate surveillance interval for monitoring the rate of aneurysmal diameter growth over time is defined on the basis of rupture risk stratification (Table 14.1) [1]:

- Very small AAAs, with DAP/DT between 3 and 3.9 cm, require reassessment every 3 years.
- Small AAAs, with DAP/DT between 4.0 and 4.9 cm, need annual follow-up.
- AAAs that reach a diameter >5.0 cm are worthy of close re-evaluation at 3–6 months.

However, the main goal is to avoid the progressive growth of the aneurysm. Lifestyle change and control of risk factors (cessation of cigarette smoking, moderate exercise, and proper diet) in association with medical therapy (antihypertensives, statins, and antiplatelet agents) are recommended as preventive measures for all patients with AAA.

A. Iannarelli (✉) · G. Trillò
Department of Diagnostic and Interventional Radiology, Santa Maria Goretti Hospital, Latina, Italy
e-mail: giovanni.trillo@uniroma1.it

Table 14.1 AAA follow-up

Maximum diameter	Recommended follow-up
Between 2.5 and 2.9 cm (ECTASIA)	Every 5 years
Between 3.0 and 3.9 cm (AAA very small)	Every 3 years
Between 4.0 and 4.9 cm (AAA small caliber)	Every 12 months
Between 5.0 and 5.4 cm (medium caliber AAA)	Every 3–6 months
≥5.5 cm (large AAA)	Vascular surgery required

Aorta with maximum diameter between 2.5 and 2.9 cm, considered as AAA (maximum size ≥1.5 times the caliber of the proximal segment)
Surgical evaluation is recommended in cases of AAA > 4.5 cm, particularly in females

The proper management of small and medium caliber AAAs (DAP/DT between 4.0 and 5.4 cm) with atherosclerotic etiology has been adequately defined in four pilot studies (UK-SAT and ADAM—[2]; CAESAR—[3]; PIVOTAL—[4]), which confirmed the effectiveness of active instrumental surveillance, as well as a significant reduction in health care expenditure. Moreover, all studies agreed on the indication for surgical treatment when a diameter ≥5.5 cm is reached or in case of rapid growth over time (>1 cm/year) and/or the onset of clinical symptoms due to AAA.

Surgical treatment is also indicated in women with AAA >4.5 cm, as a higher risk of rupture has been demonstrated.

Common opinion of these trials remains that small and medium AAAs with DAP/DT <5.5 cm should be managed conservatively, through active surveillance, also considering the prognostic factor given by the ratio of risk of rupture and risk of intra/perioperative mortality [5]. To date, as the average age and survival of the population increase, a considerable group of patients affected by AAA is not considered suitable for repair surgery, either endovascular or even less surgical, due to the comorbidities present and the low life expectancy.

Conservative Management and Follow-Up of Uncomplicated Descending Thoracic Aortic Aneurysm (DTAA) and Thoracoabdominal Aneurysm (TAAA)

The normal caliber of the thoracic aorta varies with age, sex, and body surface area (DAP/DT <3 cm) and is usually between 2.4 and 2.9 cm for the descending thoracic aorta and between 2.4 and 2.7 cm for the thoracoabdominal aorta. In general, an aneurysm (DTAA/TAAA) is defined as any increase in DAP/DT ≥50% over the normal caliber of any segment of aorta between the emergence of the left subclavian artery and its diaphragmatic hiatus (usually DAP/DT >4.0 cm). In contrast, the term dilatation/ectasia is used in cases of vessel diameters that are above normal but do not fall within the definition of aneurysm. Even in patients with a diagnosis of DTAA/TAAA, close instrumental monitoring is recommended for a correct management of the pathology, to detect possible complications early and ensure the effectiveness of medical therapy.

The adoption of rigorous protocols of instrumental surveillance is based on the evidence that uncomplicated DTAA/TAAA, managed conservatively regardless of the underlying cause, inevitably tend to grow over time with an average growth rate around 1 mm/year.

The active surveillance scheme to be observed in this type of patients is therefore based on the annual growth rate of DTAA/TAAA (reflecting the percentage of risk of rupture) and consists of an initial instrumental check at about 6 months after diagnosis, a subsequent check after an interval of 12 months, proceeding after that with annual reevaluations [6].

Other factors that influence the annual growth rate, with consequent increase in the frequency of serial controls, are represented not only by the initial diameter of the aneurysm at diagnosis, but also by the presence of imaging features with a high risk of complication/rupture (flap of dissection, intramural hematoma, ulcerated atheromasic plaque, aortitis, and penetrating trauma) and by the coexistence of connective tissue diseases (Fig. 14.1). In these cases, closer follow-up is necessary.

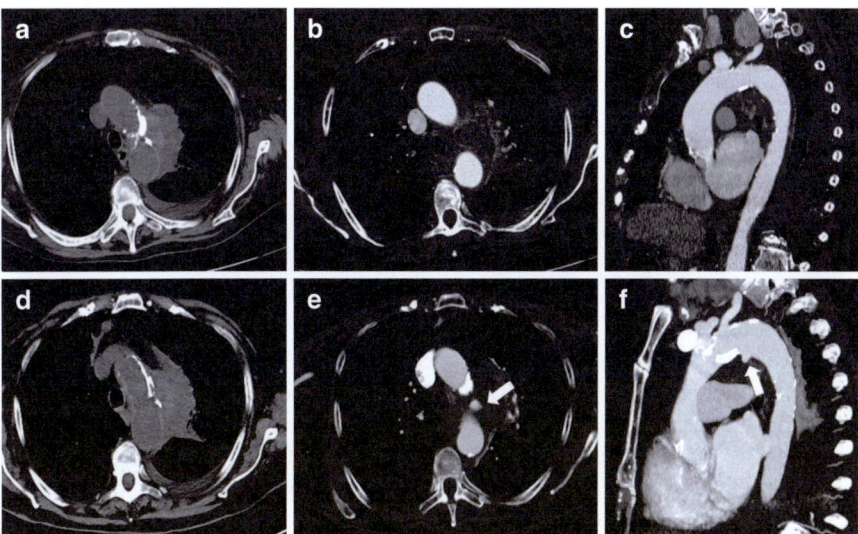

Fig. 14.1 79-years-old female admitted at the hospital for acute chest pain. CT angiography at baseline shows intramural hematoma on axial pre-contrast CT images (**a**); on the arterial phase image (**b**) and in the sagittal MIP reconstruction (**c**) the ectasia of the thoracic aorta is visible. CT re-evaluation confirms the presence of intramural hematoma (**d**); in the arterial phase is clearly visible an ulceration of the aortic wall at the level of the intramural hematoma (arrow in **e**) with small bleb of the inferior wall (arrow in **f**). The patient underwent surgical evaluation for endoprosthesis

The Role of Imaging in the Follow-Up of DTAA/TAAA and Untreated AAA

The follow-up of non-surgical aortic aneurysm pathology is mainly based on CT imaging (or MRI in case of contraindications to the first method) and ultrasound (US). It is common practice to measure the maximum diameter of the aorta in the axial plane; this is the most widely used method both for the initial diagnosis and for the implications that arise as a result of the stratification of the risk of rupture and the subsequent definition of the frequency of monitoring over time.

The need to determine minimal dimensional changes during follow-up raises the question of the accuracy and reproducibility of CT/US measurements of the axial diameter (DAP/DT) of the aorta. DAP/DT provides information only for a single segment (or rather "slice" or "section") of aneurysmal aorta. The use of modern and interesting CT imaging reconstruction algorithms allows the analysis of the total volume of the aorta in combination with the colorimetric map of the flow and its hemodynamic changes both within the aneurysm and in the various aortic segments. Such software, with very high sensitivity, allows the detection of minimal, but significant, changes in aneurysm size in the absence of significant changes in the maximum orthogonal diameter at the same level [7]. This greatly increases the observer's ability to identify which aneurysms progress over time and the efficacy of medical therapies.

There has been recent interest in assessing the trend of morphological changes, distribution, and overall volume of both intramural and endoluminal thrombotic apposition and parietal calcifications in the aneurysmal aortic tract to be monitored during follow-up [8]. These morphostructural features and their modifications over time appear to be highly correlated with the progression and risk of aneurysm rupture (Fig. 14.2), thus refining the risk category of membership and subsequent frequency of follow-up.

However, the use of morphological analysis as the only method in the management and monitoring of aneurysmal pathology of the aorta is burdened by numerous limitations, especially from a prognostic point of view: small aneurysms with a diameter similar to the initial diagnosis may vary significantly in the rate of dimensional growth over time, resulting in a probability of rupture completely different.

A more comprehensive assessment modality would allow more affidable prediction of aneurysm progression over time, with a significant reduction in the frequency of instrumental checks during follow-up.

The radiologist has a fundamental and decisive role in the follow-up of aneurysmal pathology of the aorta because he determines the evolution of the aneurysm over time helping the clinician to choose the appropriate therapeutic pathway; moreover, radiologists sensitize the patient by improving the adherence to the active surveillance program.

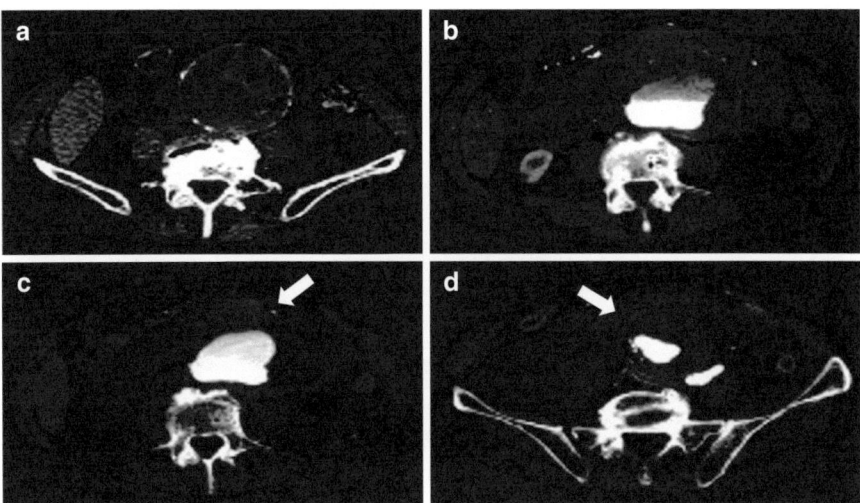

Fig. 14.2 81-years-old male with recent onset of abdominal pain and abdominal aortic aneurysm. Baseline CT scan shows hyperdense, stratified endoluminal thrombotic material, and aortic wall remodeling (**a**). During CT acquisition in arterial phase (**b–d**) is clearly visible focal defect of the anterior aortic wall with progressive leak of contrast media into the retroperitoneal space (arrow). The patient died few hours later

References

1. Moll FL, Powell JT, Fraedrich G, et al. Management of abdominal aortic aneurysms clinical practice guidelines of the European Society for Vascular Surgery. Eur J Vasc Endovasc Surg. 2011;Suppl 1:S1–S58.
2. Brown LC, Thompson SG, Greenhalgh RM, et al. Fit patients with small abdominal aortic aneurysms (AAAs) do not benefit from early intervention. J Vasc Surg. 2008;48(6):1375–81.
3. Cao P, De Rango P, Verzini F, et al. Comparison of surveillance versus aortic endo-grafting for small aneurysm repair (CAESAR): results from a randomised trial. Eur J Vasc Endovasc Surg. 2011;41(1):13–25.
4. Ouriel K. The PIVOTAL study: a randomized comparison of endovascular repair versus surveillance in patients with smaller abdominal aortic aneurysms. J Vasc Surg. 2009;49(1):266–9.
5. Wanhainen A, Verzini F, Van Herzeele I, et al. European Society for Vascular Surgery (ESVS) 2019 clinical practice guidelines on the management of abdominal aorto-iliac artery aneurysms. Eur J Vasc Endovasc Surg. 2019;57(1):8–93.
6. Riambau V, Böckler D, Brunkwall J, et al. Management of descending thoracic aorta diseases: clinical practice guidelines of the European Society for Vascular Surgery (ESVS). Eur J Vasc Endovasc Surg. 2017;53(1):4–52.
7. Moxon JV, Parr A, Emeto TI, et al. Diagnosis and monitoring of abdominal aortic aneurysm: current status and future prospects. Curr Probl Cardiol. 2010;35(10):512–48.
8. Meyrignac O, Bal L, Zadro C, et al. Combining volumetric and wall shear stress analysis from CT to assess risk of abdominal aortic aneurysm progression. Radiology. 2020;295(3):722–9.

15

Reporting Checklist: Aneurysm Follow-Up of the Abdominal Aorta

Angelo Iannarelli, Giovanni Trillò, and Valentina Romano

Untreated Aneurysm: Reporting Checklist

In patients with inoperable aortic aneurysm, angio-CT or MRI reports should mention a series of imaging features important for the further patients management.

The following is a list of the basic information to be included in the report:

- Localization (pre/post-emergence left subclavian artery, pre/post-arch section of the VI coast; supra/peri/infrarenal).
- Size (three diameters: DLxDTxDAP).
- Morphology (fusiform/sacciform).
- Diameter and length of the proximal collar (distance from the emergence of the left subclavian; distance from the emergence of the renal arteries) and the distal collar (distance from the emergence of the celiac tripod, distance from the emergence of the internal iliac arteries).
- Intravascular thrombotic load (indicating their extent relative to wall circumference) with measurement of residual lumen.
- Intramural calcifications or thromboses (indicating their extent relative to the wall circumference).
- Involvement and patency of arterial vessels emerging from the aneurysm (epi-aortic trunks, renal arteries, splanchnic arteries, accessory vessels/anatomic variants).

A. Iannarelli (✉) · G. Trillò
Department of Diagnostic and Interventional Radiology, Santa Maria Goretti Hospital, Latina, Italy
e-mail: giovanni.trillo@uniroma1.it

V. Romano
Department of Radiology, Charité Universitaetsmedizin Berlin, Berlin, Germany

© The Author(s), under exclusive license to Springer Nature Switzerland AG 2024
I. Carbone et al. (eds.), *Imaging of the Aorta*,
https://doi.org/10.1007/978-3-031-52527-8_15

- Homogeneity/unhomogeneity of peri-aneurysmal (abdominal site) loose/adipose tissue.
- Occurrence of complications (rupture, fistolization, thrombosis/embolization of downstream fragments).

In case of DTAA:

- If involving the left subclavian artery, report the caliber and dominance of the vertebral arteries.
- Describe the characteristics of the common and internal carotid arteries, in case of significant parietal atheromasic disease.

In case of AAA indicate:

- The possible involvement of the main renal arteries.
- The presence of polar/accessory renal arteries.
- The course of the renal veins (possible retroaortic).

Treated Aneurysm (Follow-Up After Evar): Reporting Checklist

1. Size (three diameters: DLxDTxDAP) of the aneurysmal sac.
2. Complications:
   (a) EARLY complications (immediate, mostly symptomatic).
      - Dissection/occlusion of iliac arteries.
      - Spurious femoral aneurysm.
      - Embolism/infarction (kidneys, intestines, and limbs).
   (b) LATE complications (can be asymptomatic, months/years after procedure).
      - Endoleak (30–40%).
      - Growth of aneurysmal sac in the absence of endoleak (endotension).
      - Formation of new aneurysms.
      - Stent-graft migration/kinking.
      - Thrombosis of the endograft.

Part V
Acute Aortic Syndrome

Acute Aortic Syndrome (AAS) and Traumatic Aortic Injury (TAI)

16

Filippo Vaccher, Davide Farina, Andrea Borghesi, and Marco Ravanelli

Intramural Hematoma (IMH)

The underlying pathophysiology of the IMH consists of the rupture of the vasa vasorum of the aorta, causing a contained hemorrhage inside the aortic wall, within the tunica media. Unlike aortic dissections, however, IMH does not interrupt the intimal layer, abutting the vessel lumen. Anyway, IMH and aortic dissection are closely related, since IMH can frequently progress into aortic dissection when the increasing IMH blood pressure "breaks" the intimal layer, opening its way into the true lumen of the vessel and creating an intimal tear from where the dissection starts and propagates. In these cases, some advocate that if the dissection is focal and very limited in extension, or if the false lumen acutely thromboses, the finding might also be described as incomplete dissection [1].

IMHs represent up to 10–30% of the AASs, manifesting with the classical symptoms of AAS (interscapular or upper back pain, hypotension and shock, syncope).

In the vast majority of cases (~90%), IMH is untriggered; in 10% of cases, instead, it has a traumatic etiology [2]. More frequently (60–70% of cases), IMH

F. Vaccher · A. Borghesi · M. Ravanelli (✉)
Institute of Radiology, Department of Medical and Surgical Specialties, Radiological Sciences, and Public Health, University of Brescia, Brescia, Italy
e-mail: andrea.borghesi@unibs.it; marco.ravanelli@unibs.it

D. Farina
Institute of Radiology, Department of Medical and Surgical Specialties, Radiological Sciences, and Public Health, University of Brescia, Brescia, Italy

Radiology Unit 2, ASST Spedali Civili di Brescia, Brescia, Italy
e-mail: davide.farina@unibs.it

involves the descending thoracic aorta (type-B IMH); involvement of the ascending aorta or the aortic arch (type-A) accounts for 10% and 30% of cases, respectively [3].

Type-A IMHs (especially those involving the ascending aorta) show worse prognosis compared to type-B ones. Over time, the range of possible evolutions of IMH is quite high. Spontaneous healing through fibrous scar formation occurs in 34% of cases, progression to penetrating aortic ulcer and dissection is seen in 16–47% of cases, namely 14% of those involving the descending aorta and 88% of those in the ascending aorta. Aortic rupture occurs in 20–45% of cases.

Imaging

CT angiography (CTA) is the imaging technique of choice for the diagnosis of IMHs with sensitivity reaching 96% [3]. MR angiography (MRA) is far less convenient in the acute phase, because of issues related to availability, acquisition times, and clinical monitoring of hemodynamically unstable patients.

CTA displays a hyperdense parietal thickening (>5 mm) with a circumferential or, more frequently, crescent-shaped morphology. IMH's spontaneous hyperintensity is better identified at unenhanced CTA images, when viewed with a narrow window level (e.g., window width 200 HU, center level 40 HU). Thick sections (5 mm) examination could be helpful, because of an increased signal/noise ratio [4] (Fig. 16.1).

On MRI, IMH manifests as a spontaneously T1w hyperintense signal in the aortic wall due to the presence of methaemoglobin. In selected case, this can be of help for the differential diagnosis with other entities, as aortitis, which displays T1w hypointensity due to parietal edema of the aortic wall (Fig. 16.2).

IMH generally involves a long segment of the aortic wall, with straight craniocaudal progression, unlike thrombosed false lumens in aortic dissections, which progress spiraling along the vessel wall.

When an IMH develops, aortic luminal diameter is focally reduced, with a clearly identifiable transition point (better recognized in parasagittal multiplanar reconstruction series). This morphologic detail helps to distinguish IMH from other conditions, like aortitis and atherosclerosis which induce parietal thickening while preserving the effective luminal diameter.

In addition, IMH-related parietal thickening causes displacement of any intimal calcification toward the aortic lumen; atherosclerotic wall plaques, instead, develop on the luminal side, moving intimal calcifications outwards.

Generally, there is no measurable enhancement within the aortic wall (helping in differential diagnosis with inflammatory wall thickening). Anyway, Ulcer Like Projections (ULPs: finger-like projections in the thickened wall, opacified by contrast medium) are a common finding: they usually develop over time and depict a connection between the aortic lumen and pouch-like ulcerations of the thickened, pathologic aortic wall of the IMH. Similarly, *Intramural Blood Pools* (IBPs) can be encountered, seen as a focal pool of enhancement within the IMH, with no connection to the aortic blood pool: they arise from restricted bleeding or pseudoaneurysm

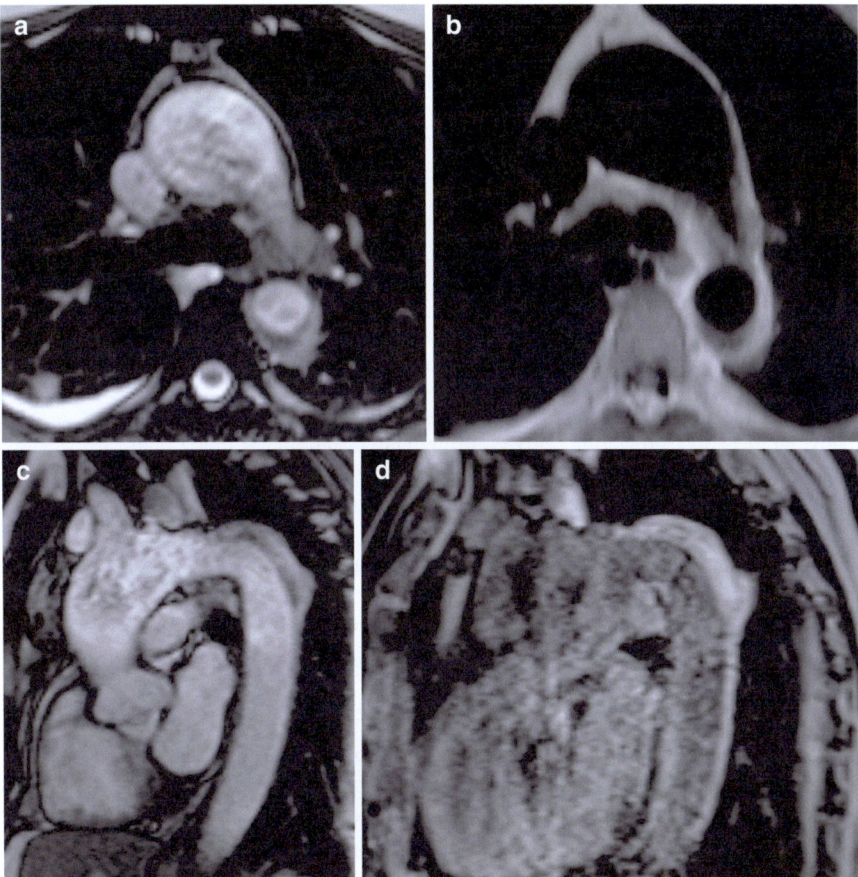

Fig. 16.1 Unenhanced MRI images of IMH of the aortic isthmus and descending thoracic aorta. The aortic wall is thickened, with intermediate MR signal in the axial (**a**) and parasagittal (**c**) True-FISP hybrid sequences. Signal hypointensity in T2-weighted sequences (**b**) and T1-hyperintense signal in T1 fat-sat sequences (**d**) are indicative of IMH

formation of small aortic side branches (intercostal arteries, lumbar arteries, and bronchial arteries), arising from the segment involved by the IMH. Both ULPs and IBPs should be considered signs suggesting of impending evolution of the IMH to penetrating ulcer or dissection [1].

Treatment and Evolution in Time

Similarly to what happens in the aortic dissection, Stanford classification is the basis of IMH management. Type-A IMH has an overall mortality rate of 39.1%, increasing proportionally with the proximity of the segment involved to the aortic root [5].

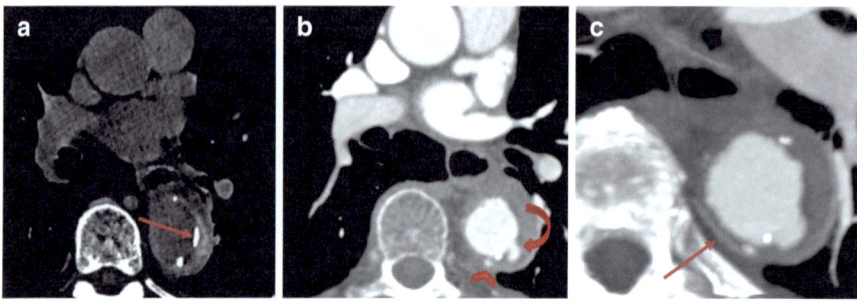

Fig. 16.2 Intramural hematoma with spontaneous wall hyperdensity of the aortic wall on unenhanced CT scans (**a**) and displacement towards the aortic lumen of intimal calcifications (arrow). In the same patient, on CTA (**b**), two focal opacities by contrast medium in intramural pools of enhancement within the thickness of the IMH: these represent, respectively, an ulcer-like projection (curved arrow) and an intramural blood pool (arrowhead), respectively, supplied by a posterior intercostal artery, as evident from MIP reconstructions (**c**, arrow)

In such cases, aortic surgery is indicated (open repair, OR) by most of the current guidelines [3]. Some studies and some recent guidelines (such as the Japanese Circulation Society Guidelines; [1]) suggest a conservative management of type-A IMH, leaving delayed surgical approach for those patients developing complications. In these series, however, delayed surgical approach carries a slightly higher mortality rate (14% vs. 10%) and an overall intervention rate still as high as 45%. In addition, the need of a closer follow-up protocol in these patients, implies higher costs and higher radiation exposure [4].

Type-B IMH has a reported mortality rate of 8.3% [5]. In these cases, a conservative treatment with close follow-up is advised, unless clinical or radiological signs of complication arise. In the case of high-risk type-B IMH, endovascular approach (TEVAR) is the gold standard [6]. The risk of IMH progression, especially in type-B, is heralded by the following clinical and radiological signs:

- Parietal thickness >11 mm at diagnosis;
- Presence of ULPs or IBPs;
- Initial signs of enhancement within the parietal thickness of the IMH;
- Overall aortic diameter >55 mm in type-A or >40 mm in type-B;
- Aortic diameter rapidly increasing in time (>1 cm/year);
- Sings of impending rupture such as hemopericardium/pericardial effusion, hemothorax/pleural effusion, periaortic fat stranding or periaortic hematoma;
- Clinical worrisome signs (pain, hemodynamic instability).

Endovascular repair of IMH requires the use of long stent grafts, in order to adequately seal the aortic lumen in a point where the vessel wall returns normal [7]. For this reason, in patients with unsuitable aortic anatomy or extreme landing zones for endovascular devices, OR should be preferred.

Penetrating Atherosclerotic Ulcer (PAU)

PAU is one of the possible complications of advanced atherosclerotic disease; it consists of the deep ulceration at the surface of an atherosclerotic plaque, eroding the vessel wall up to the internal elastic lamina and the medial layer. The process generally modifies the straight silhouette of the external aortic profile. PAU should be carefully differentiated from an ulcerated atherosclerotic plaque, since the latter shows only superficial ulceration, limited to the thickness of the plaque with no extension to the intimal and medial layer. In addition, ulcerated plaques do not modify the local external aortic contour.

In approximately 80% of cases, PAU is associated with IMH of the nearby aortic segments, both upstream and downstream, with varying degree of extension [5].

PAUs represent 2–7% of all cases of AASs and manifest with classical symptoms, mirroring those of IMH. In up to 20% of the diagnosed cases, anyway, PAUs is an incidental finding in patients showing no suggesting clinical signs or symptoms, often scanned for completely different conditions.

Over 23% of PAUs progress over time to extensive IMH, dissection, saccular aneurysm, aortic wall pseudoaneurysm and, ultimately, to frank aortic rupture. The percentage of PAU progressing to complication is higher for symptomatic patients (43%) than asymptomatic ones (17%). Due to its atherosclerotic nature, PAU can also cause distal embolization of atherosclerotic debris with end-organ ischemia [5].

Imaging

Commonly, PAU is seen on cross-sectional imaging as a contrast-filled pouch with a "crater-like" appearance, developing within the context of an atherosclerotic parietal plaque and protruding from the external surface of the aortic wall. This pouch has neck connecting with the aortic lumen, with variable width and depth (Fig. 16.3). The internal aortic profile appears thickened, hypodense, and irregular due to the presence of unstable atherosclerotic plaques. Unlike IMH and aortic dissection, PAU is by definition a focal lesion, affecting a short segment of the aorta; however, as atherosclerosis is a diffuse disease, PAU is frequently multifocal (Fig. 16.4). The most frequent location for a PAU is in the distal descending thoracic aorta (61.2%), followed by the abdominal aorta (29.7%). Less commonly PAU involves the aortic arch, whereas only in rare cases it is found in the ascending aorta.

IMH frequently develops as a consequence of PAU progression on upstream and downstream aortic segments, with varying extension: unlike PAU, anyway, IMH displays a thickened wall but with regular and smooth internal and external aortic contour.

Chronic PAU (those most frequently diagnosed as incidental findings in asymptomatic patients) may be partially or completely thrombosed. PAU degenerated to dissection, instead, frequently display a thickened intimal flap (often with intimal calcifications and parietal plaques) extending proximally to the PAU location for a

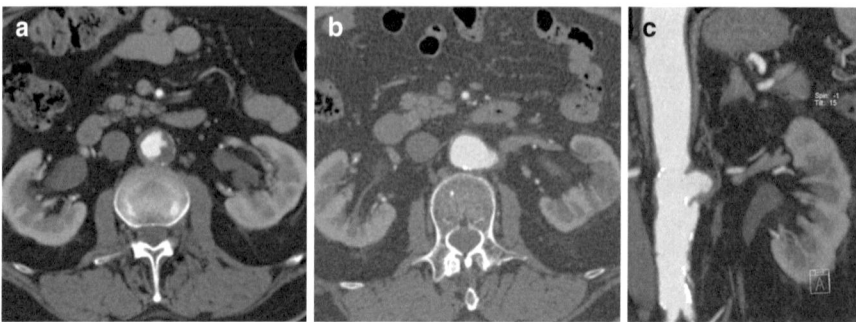

Fig. 16.3 PAUs is often manifest as a complication of advanced atherosclerosis: evolution over time from unstable ulcerated atheromasic atherosclerotic plaque (**a**) to PAU (**b**) with involvement of the elastic lamina of the vessel and alteration of the external aortic profile, evident in MPR paracoronal reconstructions (**c**)

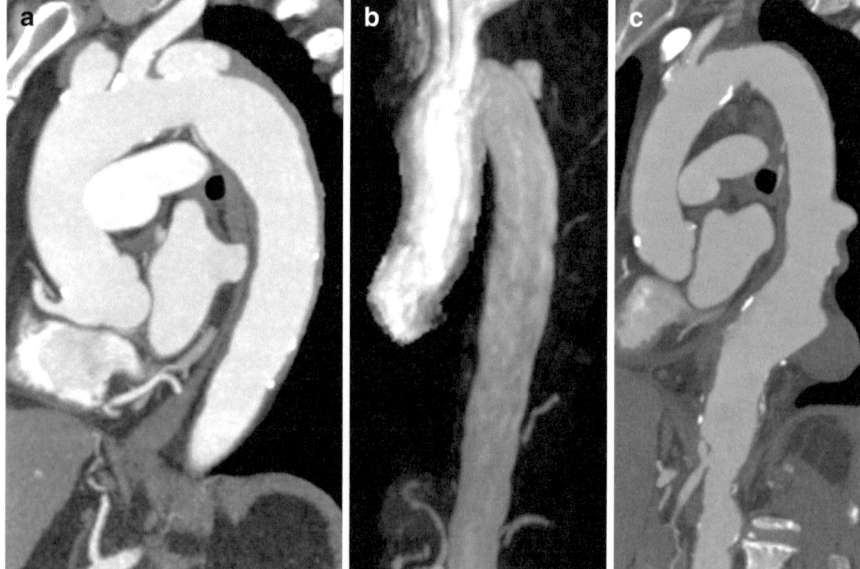

Fig. 16.4 Parasagittal MIP angio-CT Angiography (**a**) and angio-MR Angiography (**b**) reconstructions in two patients with PAUs of the aortic isthmus with classic "peptic ulcer" appearance. Parasagittal MIP reconstructions angio-CT of CTA reconstructions (**c**) in a patient with advanced atherosclerosis and, multifocal PAUs of the descending aorta, some of them chronic and partially thrombosed

couple of centimeters. These findings help in the differential diagnosis with classical type-B dissection, characterized by a thin intimal flap, extending distally from the intimal tear and for quite a long tract [2].

For the reasons already discussed for IMH, CTA is the technique of choice in patients with AAS; MRI more commonly identifies incidentally found PAU. Besides providing the diagnosis, both the techniques identify any related complication or "at-risk" feature and offer all the anatomic details that guide the surgical planning.

Treatment and Evolution in Time

PAU of the ascending aorta is extremely rare, but invariably progresses to aortic rupture, requiring surgical treatment [3, 7]. PAUs located in the descending aorta, instead, can be managed conservatively, especially if accidentally encountered in asymptomatic patients and classified as "low-risk" PAUs [5].

The clinical and radiological features of "high-risk" PAUs described in literature [3, 6, 8, 9] are:

- typical AAS symptoms, including pain, hemodynamic instability, signs of distal embolization;
- presence of associated IMH;
- significative depth of the ulceration or longitudinal extension (>20 mm);
- width of the neck connecting with the aortic lumen >10 mm;
- significant increase in size or morphologic modification during follow-up;
- increased aortic diameter in the involved aortic region (>55 mm in the ascending aorta; >40 mm in the descending aorta);
- signs of impending aortic rupture, pericardial effusion, increasing pleural effusion, periaortic hematoma.

The prevalence of critical scenarios in patients with symptomatic PAUs, anyway, is notably higher than in those with type-B dissection (risk of aortic rupture, respectively, of 40% in PAU vs. 7% and 4% in type-A and type-B dissections; [10]). For these reasons, follow-up is mandatory, especially during the first month from diagnosis. Then, the radiological follow-up is suggested every 3 months in the first year, every 6 months during the second and third year, and, thereafter, yearly [8].

TEVAR is the treatment of choice for high-risk PAUs if the patient meets the anatomic criteria for the feasibility of the procedure (suitable vascular access, adequate proximal and distal neck length, low grade vessel tortuosity) (Fig. 16.5). With this approach, perioperative mortality rate is 4.8%, compared to 16% of OR [5, 11].

PAU with associated extensive IMH are deemed at risk of TEVAR failure, because the metallic barbs and anchors of the endovascular graft might damage the intimal layer in a segment of diseased vessel, exposing a weakened and thrombosed medial layer and leading to a dissection. In these cases, extensive aortic coverage is indicated, with device landing on unaffected aortic wall. If not feasible, OR conversion is suggested.

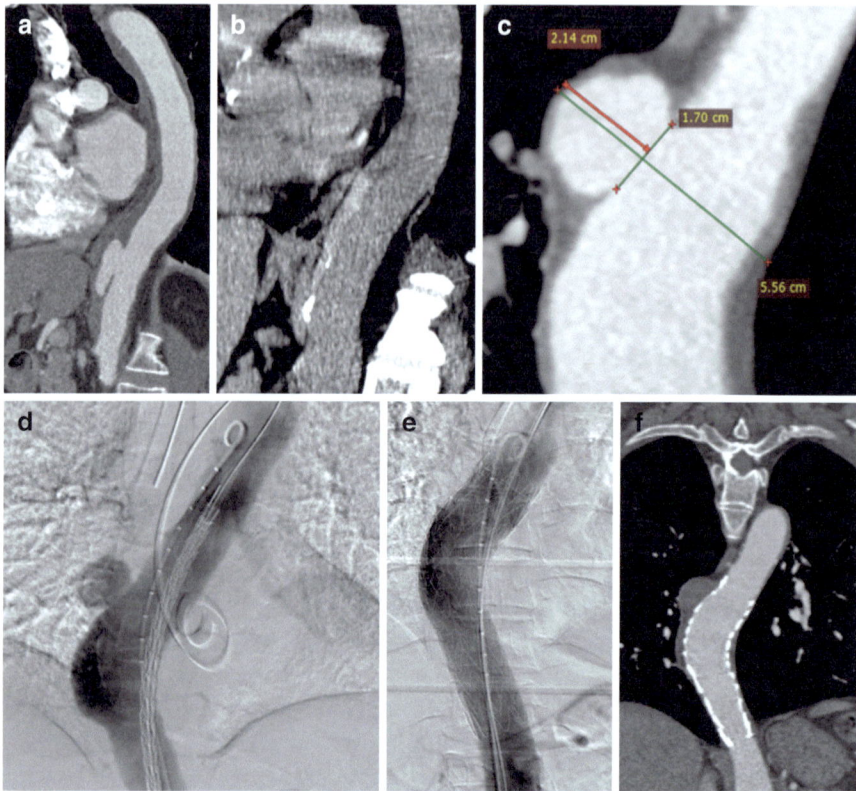

Fig. 16.5 Radiological "at risk features" characteristics in a patient with a PAU of the abdominal aorta (**a**) and associated extensive upstream and downstream IMH, spontaneously hyperdense on unenhanced CT scans (**b**). Another high-risk thoracic PAU (**c**) according to the criteria of ulcer depth, maximum aortic diameter and collar width. Relief features confirmed by the subsequent diagnostic angiography (**d**) and successfully treated by TEVAR. Complete exclusion of PAU from the circulation demonstrated by at the intraoperative final angiography (**e**) and at the post-operative control CT angiography (**f**)

Traumatic Aortic Injury (TAI)

Traumatic aortic injury (TAI) is a life-threatening, time-sensitive condition occurring as a consequence of blunt trauma or penetrating injury, most often in the setting of car or motor vehicle accidents with steep deceleration (>50%) after frontal or lateral impact (70–85%). Among the spectrum TAI, traumatic aortic rupture (TAR) is the most severe lesion, consisting of a complete or near-complete damage of the aortic wall. TAR is a rare event with extremely high mortality rates (reaching 80–90%) [12].

Several pathogenic mechanisms are considered responsible of TAI: torque mechanism, "water-hammer" effect (with sudden obstruction of blood flow due to thoracic compression and increased radial pressure on vessel walls), "osseous pinch" of the vessel between thoracic spine and sternal bone, deceleration-induced tearing forces on aortic points of fixation (aortic isthmus and ligamentum arteriosum).

Clinical signs and symptoms suggestive of TAI in trauma patients include: peripheric hypotension, possibly with upper limbs hypertension, deep thoracic lacerations, asymmetric peripheral pulses, hemodynamic instability.

Imaging

TAI may occur in any segment of the aorta; however, the most commonly involved sites are the less mobile tracts, i.e., the aortic root, isthmus—near the ligamentum arteriosum— diaphragmatic segment. TAI located at the aortic root has the highest mortality rate, with only a minority of patients reaching the CT room (5–10%). The isthmus is the most frequent location (95% in the surgical series; 65% in the autoptic ones) and the lesion is usually located along the infero-medial profile of the distal aortic arch and/or the antero-medial portion of the isthmus. Only a small number of TAI extends to the origin of the epiaortic vessels (4%) [13].

In patients with TAR, several other traumatic lesions are invariably present: multiple rib fractures (75%), abdominal organ injury or diaphragmatic injury (74%), concussion (52%), single or multiple fracture of the pelvis (40%), spine fractures, cardiac injury.

Radiological findings suggestive of TAI can be divided into direct and indirect. Direct findings include intimal flap, IMH, endoluminal thrombotic apposition, pseudoaneurysm formation, and contrast medium extravasation, more commonly contained by perivascular hematoma.

Indirect radiological signs of TAI include: periaortic hematoma, abrupt variation in aortic caliber (aortic pseudocoarctation), abnormal external aortic contour, hemothorax, and/or hemopericardium (Fig. 16.6).

In a patient with a history of recent traumatic event, the detection of a mediastinal hematoma should always raise the suspect of possible TAI: generally, if a subtle line of adipose tissue separates the hematoma from the aorta, TAI is unlikely. However, it must be emphasized that the absence of a mediastinal hematoma does not rule out the presence of a TAIs; more than 20% of low grade TAI is not associated with the presence of a mediastinal/periaortic hematoma [14].

A consensus-based classification of the severity of TAIs was produced [15], taking into account not only radiological findings, but also prognostic indicators and patient's management suggestions. Four degrees of increasing severity were described (Fig. 16.7):

- Grade 1: (10%), corresponds to the so-called minimal aortic injury (MAI) [13]; it is an isolated intimal injury (intimal flap or intimal thrombotic appositions), with longitudinal extension along the vessel <1 cm and no external aortic contour abnormality.

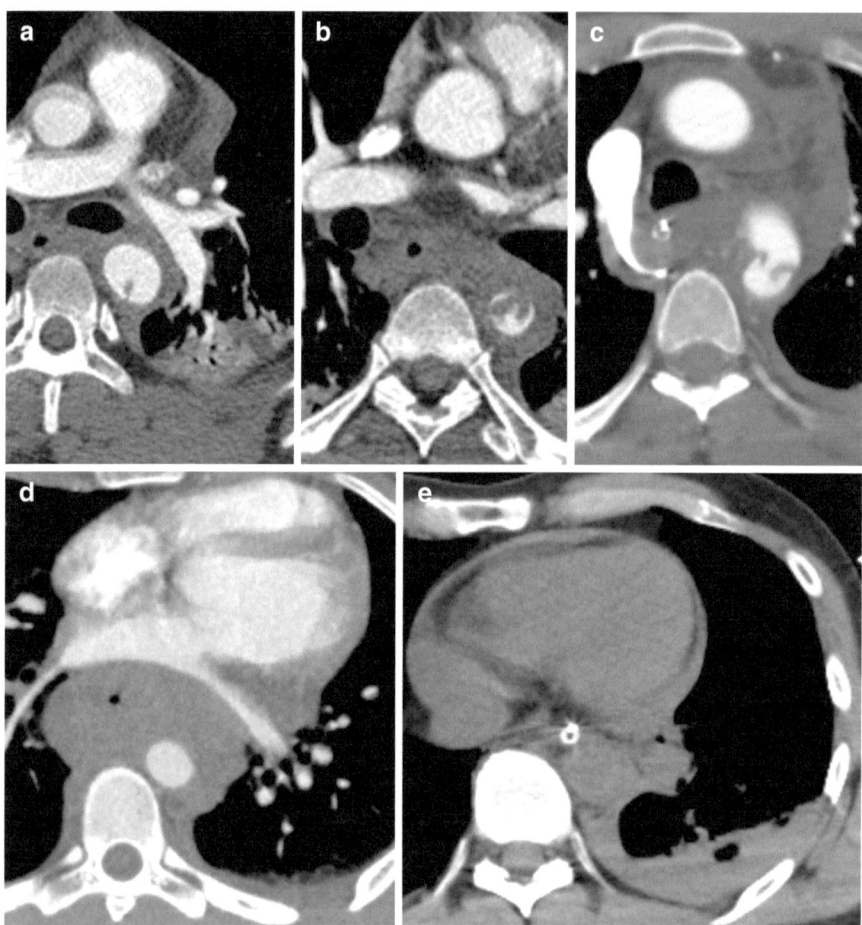

Fig. 16.6 Direct and indirect CT signs in patients with TAI. Intimal flap in a minimal aortic injury (**a**); endoluminal thrombosis of the intimal flap (**b**); abrupt reduction of aortic caliber at the isthmus to be referred to in keeping with pseudocoarctation (**c**); voluminous periaortic hematoma in the mediastinum, resulting in compression of the pulmonary veins (**d**); hemopericardium and hemothorax in a patient after motor vehicle trauma (**e**)

- Grade 2: is an injury involving the medial layer (IMH or dissection) or an isolated intimal layer injury (intimal flap or intimal thrombotic appositions) with longitudinal extension >1 cm. No external aortic contour abnormality can be identified.
- Grade 3: is a sub-adventitial damage of the vessel wall (e.g., pseudoaneurysm formation) causing a bulging/alteration of the normal external aortic profile.
- Grade 4: traumatic injury extending through all the thickness of the aortic wall, from the intima to the adventitial layer (e.g., aortic rupture with active bleeding or circumferential aortic rupture with contained bleeding). It is the case of the previously mentioned TAR.

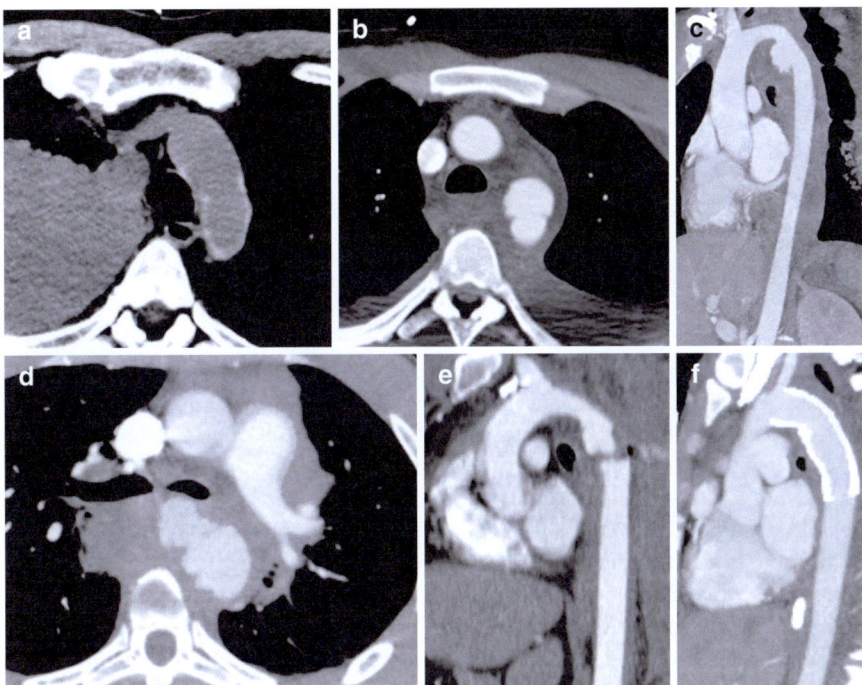

Fig. 16.7 Grade II TAI (**a**) with intramural arch hematoma of the aortic arch extended with extension to the descending aorta, without alteration of the external aortic profile. In grade III TAI the damage is sub-adventitial with alteration of the external aortic profile evidence of external aortic contour abnormality, as in the post-traumatic pseudoaneurysm of the isthmus visible in the axial (**b**) and parasagittal (**c**) planes. Grade IV TAI refers to complete parietal damage, with active spread of mdc in the mediastinum (**d**) or circumferential aortic rupture (**e**). The patient with aortic transection (**e**) was efficaciously treated with TEVAR, as demonstrated by the follow-up CT scan (**f**)

Diagnostic sensitivity is crucial for any diagnostic technique applied to TAI investigation, given the fact that mortality rates at 4 months in misdiagnosed TAI reach 90% [12].

CTA is considered the diagnostic modality of choice in TAI, with reported diagnostic sensitivity of 96% and a specificity reaching 99% [16].

MRA is of little use in the acute setting. It is reserved to hemodynamically stable patients, with doubtful or minimal injuries requiring serial monitoring, in order to reduce the radiation exposure in an overall young group of patients.

Chest radiography is executed in the majority of cases in the emergency setting, to verify the positioning of various medical devices (e.g., endotracheal tube) and to rule out emergencies in need of prompt medical treatment (e.g., extensive pneumothorax or massive hemothorax). Although chest radiography has low sensitivity and specificity, some radiological red flags should alert the radiologist of a possible TAI. These mainly include a widening of the mediastinum, which may be focal at the aortopulmonary window—associated with loss of its normal concavity—or generalized (>6 cm width in standing radiographic examination and >6 cm or width or >25% of the overall chest width in the supine patient). Additional findings include the rightwards tracheal shift and the downward dislocation of the right main bronchus.

Diagnostic Pitfalls in TAI

Particular attention should be made to some infrequent radiological findings, which could be mistaken for acute aortic pathology and TAI.

- Ductus diverticulum: persistence of a residual diverticular remnant of the ductus arteriosus, seen as an irregularity of the aortic wall at the isthmus, along the inferior profile. In the fetal circulation, the ductus arteriosus connects the pulmonary artery with the systemic arterial circulation, resulting in a functional bypass of the pulmonary circulation. The ductus diverticulum displays regular contours, with no abnormality of the periaortic tissues. It has an obtuse insertion angle on the aortic wall and may have calcifications along its intimal profile, as opposed to TAI, which displays periaortic tissue inhomogeneity, has no local intimal calcifications and forms an acute angle of insertion on the aortic wall.
- Aortic branch vessels infundibulum: it is a focal irregularity of the outer aortic profile, corresponding to a dilation at the ostium of some aortic branch vessels (e.g., intercostal arteries, bronchial arteries, and brachiocephalic artery). It can be recognized by its conic, triangular shape, with smooth margins and by the presence of a branch vessel originating from its apex. In the setting of acute trauma, such infundibulum may be misinterpreted as a pseudoaneurysm.
- Pulsation artifacts along the proximal ascending aorta: these can mimic a dissection. Repetition of the CTA with ECG-gated or non-cardiac-synchronized high-pitch acquisition may be necessary to rule out the differential diagnosis.
- Hemiazygos vein opacification: hemiazygos vein runs posteriorly and laterally to the descending aorta and can be opacified in the arterial phase due to retrograde filling with high flow-rate injections. In some cases, it may mimic an irregularity of the aortic contour; following the vessel course is crucial for the differential diagnosis.
- Pericardial recess: a cranial extension of the pericardial sac along the proximal ascending aorta may be misinterpreted as an IMH or mediastinal hematoma. The homogeneous fluid density measured in the pericardial recess generally solves the differential diagnosis.

Treatment and Evolution in Time

Patient's management depends on the severity of the findings.

A mediastinal hematoma in the absence of any sign of aortic rupture can be handled conservatively, with CTA follow-up scans at 48–72 h or conclusive evaluation with trans-esophageal echocardiography [14].

Similarly, MAI (grade 1 injury) can be managed conservatively, with close follow-up with imaging [5, 15]. However, currently there is no agreement on the timing of the radiological follow-up, especially in the first period.

Increasing evidence is suggesting the efficacy of conservative management also in grade 2 aortic injuries [5, 14]. This explains why the most clinically oriented classifications of TAI [17], classify grade 1 and 2 injuries in a single category of category of TAIs, characterized by the absence of abnormalities of the external aortic contour.

Grade 3 and 4 TAIs, on the other hand, should promptly (within 24 h) undergo surgical/endovascular treatment [15]. Delay in the operative management, however, may be unavoidable in patients with other severe injuries, requiring urgent treatment (e.g., cranio-facial trauma) [18].

OR is strongly advised for lesions involving the ascending aorta or the aortic arch. Endovascular repair (TEVAR), however, has gained increasing importance over time because of the lower operative mortality rates (9% vs. 19%) and lower risk of paraplegia and perioperative complications (9% vs. 22%) [19].

TEVAR is considered the treatment of choice for TAI involving aortic segments from the isthmus onward, in the presence of a favorable aortic anatomy. Cross-sectional imaging techniques provided detailed representation of the course, diameter and walls of the aorta. However, some additional facts should be taken into account: oversizing of the aortic prosthetic device of 10–15% is advised, with a minimum aortic diameter of 22 mm; length of coverage greater than the aortic lesion (at least 4 cm) should be attempted; proximal sealing zone of 10 mm. In this light, when facing a TAI located at the aortic isthmus (most common scenario), the radiologist should try to describe the aortic diameter proximally and distally to the TAI, the length of TAI extension and its relative position with respect to the left subclavian artery. In addition, in the event of an unfavorable proximal landing zone with likely coverage of the left subclavian artery, the vertebral arteries should be examined (normal/abnormal origin, patency, dominance).

The presence of any vascular anomaly or aorto-coronary bypass grafts should also be mentioned, together with any possible difficulties regarding vascular access point (femoral, brachial) included in the examination.

Any injury to the epiaortic vessels associated to TAI is mandatory of OR with sternotomy and vascular exposure (Fig. 16.8).

TAI requires long-term follow-up to ensure the prosthetic graft durability. Particular attention should be reserved to young patients treated with TEVAR, because of physiologic aortic growth and modification with risks of endoleak

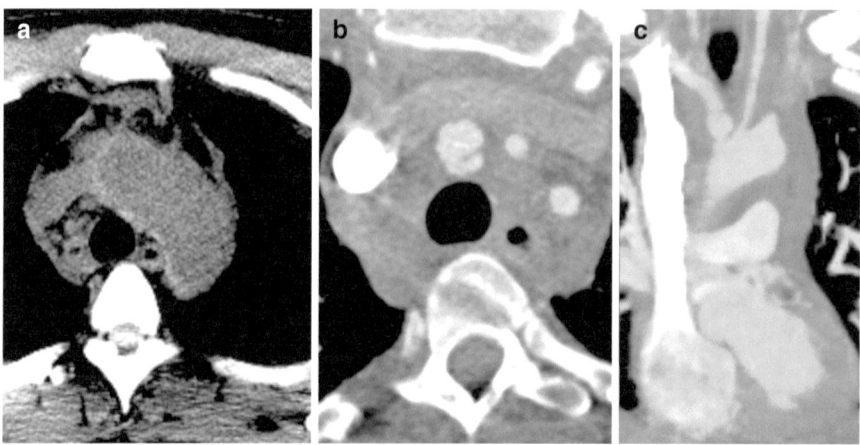

Fig. 16.8 Traumatic lesions of the aortic arch with involvement of the epiaortic vessels are less frequent and require open intervention OR. A Patient with grade II TAI classified as grade II for the presence of extensive IMH of the aortic arch (**a**), with a pseudoaneurysm of the proximal section of the innominate artery (**b**), also visible in the paracoronal MIP reconstructions (**c**). The patient was treated with OR in which de-branching and bridging of the supra-aortic trunks was performed

development, graft failure, coarctation and aneurismatic degeneration of the injured vessel in the long run. In this long-lasting follow-up, MRA might play a role, achieving a significant reduction in radiation exposure for these patients.

References

1. Vilacosta I, San Román J, di Bartolomeo R, et al. Acute aortic syndrome revisited. J Am Coll Cardiol. 2021;78(21):2106–25.
2. Dore R, Zompatori M, Magnaldi S. Manuale di tomografia computerizzata multidetettore. Milano: Poletto Editore; 2008.
3. Bossone E, LaBounty TM, Eagle KA. Acute aortic syndromes: diagnosis and management, an update. Eur Heart J. 2018;39(9):739–49d.
4. Gutschow SE, Walker CM, Martínez-Jiménez S, et al. Emerging concepts in intramural hematoma imaging. Radiographics. 2016;36(3):660–74.
5. Cronenwett JL, Johnston KW, Rutherford RB, editors. Rutherford's vascular surgery. 6th ed. Philadelphia, PA: Elsevier/Saunders; 2005.
6. Spanos K, Kölbel T, Giannoukas AD. Current trends in aortic intramural hematoma management-a shift from conservative to a more aggressive treatment. Ann Cardiothorac Surg. 2019;8(4):497–9.
7. Eggebrecht H, Plicht B, Kahlert P, et al. Intramural hematoma and penetrating ulcers: indications to endovascular treatment. Eur J Vasc Endovasc Surg. 2009;38(6):659–65.
8. Evangelista A, Maldonado G, Moral S, et al. Intramural hematoma and penetrating ulcer in the descending aorta: differences and similarities. Ann Cardiothorac Surg. 2019;8(4):456–70.
9. Nathan DP, Boonn W, Lai E, et al. Presentation, complications, and natural history of penetrating atherosclerotic ulcer disease. J Vasc Surg. 2012;55(1):10–5.
10. Hayashi H, Matsuoka Y, Sakamoto I, et al. Penetrating atherosclerotic ulcer of the aorta: imaging features and disease concept. Radiographics. 2000;20(4):995–1005.

11. D'Annoville T, Ozdemir BA, Alric P, et al. Thoracic endovascular aortic repair for penetrating aortic ulcer: literature review. Ann Thorac Surg. 2016;101(6):2272–8.
12. Cullen EL, Lantz EJ, Johnson CM, et al. Traumatic aortic injury: CT findings, mimics, and therapeutic options. Cardiovasc Diagn Ther. 2014;4(3):238–44.
13. Steenburg SD, Ravenel JG. Acute traumatic thoracic aortic injuries: experience with 64-MDCT. AJR Am J Roentgenol. 2008;191(5):1564–9.
14. Rajput MZ, Raptis DA, Raptis CA, et al. Imaging of acute traumatic aortic injury. Curr Radiol Rep. 2018;6(6):19.
15. Lee WA, Matsumura JS, Mitchell RS, et al. Endovascular repair of traumatic thoracic aortic injury: clinical practice guidelines of the Society for Vascular Surgery. J Vasc Surg. 2011;53(1):187–92.
16. Steenburg SD, Ravenel JG, Ikonomidis JS, et al. Acute traumatic aortic injury: imaging evaluation and management. Radiology. 2008;248(3):748–62.
17. Lamarche Y, Berger FH, Nicolaou S, et al. Vancouver simplified grading system with computed tomographic angiography for blunt aortic injury. J Thorac Cardiovasc Surg. 2012;144(2):347–54, 354.e1.
18. Fox N, Schwartz D, Salazar JH, et al. Evaluation and management of blunt traumatic aortic injury: a practice management guideline from the Eastern Association for the Surgery of Trauma. J Trauma Acute Care Surg. 2015;78(1):136–46.
19. Andersen ND, Williams JB, Hanna JM, et al. Results with an algorithmic approach to hybrid repair of the aortic arch. J Vasc Surg. 2013;57(3):655–67.

Aortic Dissection: Imaging and Elements of Endovascular Pretreatment Evaluation

17

Nicolò Schicchi, Matteo Marcucci, Paolo Esposto Pirani, Marco Fogante, Fatjon Cela, and Liliana Balardi

Diagnostic Framework

Aortic dissection (AD) occurs when blood enters the medial layer of the aortic wall through a tear or penetrating ulcer in the intima and tracks longitudinally along with the media, forming an intimal flap and a second blood-filled channel (false lumen) within the vessel wall. The intima may further tear, creating a re-entry breach for blood flow into the true lumen, with a mixing of the blood flow between the true and false lumen. This promotes a rebalancing of the flows, which allows depressurization of the false lumen.

AD can be spontaneous, iatrogenic or traumatic.

In relation to the time of onset, it is classified as:

- hyperacute: <24 h;
- acute: 2–7 days;

N. Schicchi (✉)
SOS Diagnostica Radiologica Cardiovascolare, Azienda Ospedaliero Universitaria "Ospedali Riuniti", Ancona, Italy
e-mail: nicolo.schicchi@ospedaliriuniti.marche.it

M. Marcucci
U.O.C. di Radiodiagnostica, Ospedale Generale Provinciale di Macerata, Macerata, Italy

P. E. Pirani · M. Fogante · F. Cela
SOD Materno-Infantile, Senologica, Cardiologica ed Ecografica Ambulatoriale, Azienda Ospedaliero Universitaria "Ospedali Riuniti", Ancona, Italy
e-mail: paolo.espostopirani@ospedaliriuniti.marche.it; marco.fogante@ospedaliriuniti.marche.it; fation.cela@ospedaliriuniti.marche.it

L. Balardi
Azienda Ospedaliero Universitaria "Ospedali Riuniti", Ancona, Italy
e-mail: liliana.balardi@ospedaliriuniti.marche.it

© The Author(s), under exclusive license to Springer Nature Switzerland AG 2024
I. Carbone et al. (eds.), *Imaging of the Aorta*,
https://doi.org/10.1007/978-3-031-52527-8_17

Table 17.1 Aortic dissection: classifications of DeBakey and Stanford

DeBakey		Stanford
Type I	Ascending, arch, thoracic aorta	Ascending, with or without involvement of the descending thoracic aorta
Type II	Ascending aorta only	
Type III a	Descending aorta after the origin of the left subclavian, limited to the thoracic	Descending after the origin of the left subclavian
Type III b	Descending aorta after the origin of the left subclavian, extended to the abdominal	

– subacute: 8–30 days;
– chronic: ≥30 days.

In relation to the location and extension, the most widely used classifications are those of DeBakey and Stanford, given in Table 17.1.

Basically, Stanford's type A includes DeBakey's types I and II, while Stanford's type B includes DeBakey's types IIIa and IIIb.

The Stanford classification is widely used because it guides the therapeutic choice: type A dissection often requires urgent surgical treatment; type B dissection is generally treated conservatively-pharmacologically. The main purpose of imaging in AD is the complete evaluation of the entire aorta, including aortic diameters, the extent of the flap of dissection, the relationship with adjacent anatomical structures, the presence of parietal thrombosis, and the possible involvement in the dissection process of the aortic valve or splanchnic branches with low organ vascularization [1].

Computed tomography angiography (CTA), magnetic resonance imaging (MRI), and echocardiography are useful methods to confirm or exclude the diagnosis of AD. However, CT and MRI are superior to echocardiography in assessing the extent and involvement of aortic branches [2]. Echocardiography can be used in hemodynamically unstable patient, to monitor the patient in the operating room and in the postoperative intensive care unit. Chest X-ray (CXR) may be considered when the patient is hemodynamically stable and has a low pre-test probability of AD based on clinical data. Aortography is predominantly used with therapeutic findings, particularly during the procedure of repair by positioning endoprosthesis [3].

Radiological Signs of Aortic Dissection

The main sign of AD on CTA is the presence of the intimal flap floating in the aortic lumen caused by the disconnection of the intimal layer and the elastic lamina of the middle arterial layer from the residual aortic wall. This lesion promotes progressive longitudinal dissection of the vessel layers with the creation of two lumens that spiral around each other. In the affected section of abdominal aorta, an intimal breach may be visible creating a re-entry tear for blood flow into the true lumen (Fig. 17.1).

17 Aortic Dissection: Imaging and Elements of Endovascular Pretreatment Evaluation

The correct identification of the "true lumen" and the "false lumen" is mandatory to clarify which collaterals are exclusively perfused by the false lumen and for a subsequent endovascular therapeutic planning (Table 17.2). The true lumen is in continuity with the non-dissected portion of the aorta and generally presents smaller dimensions because it is compressed by the false lumen. The true lumen is surrounded by calcifications of the outer wall (if present) (Fig. 17.2). In contrast, the false lumen is larger, with a characteristically lower contrast density than the true lumen, due to a slower enhancement. In the case of chronic dissection, the false lumen is commonly thrombosed and does not present a significant enhancement. In addition, the false lumen is characterized by the "beak sign": the false lumen wedges around the true lumen, due to permanent systolic pressure, with the formation of an acute angle between the mid-intimal flap and the residual mid-adventitial lamina on the aortic wall (Fig. 17.3). In many cases, a "spider's web sign" is observed for the presence of thin collagen filaments and shoots proper to the middle layer within the false lumen (Fig. 17.3).

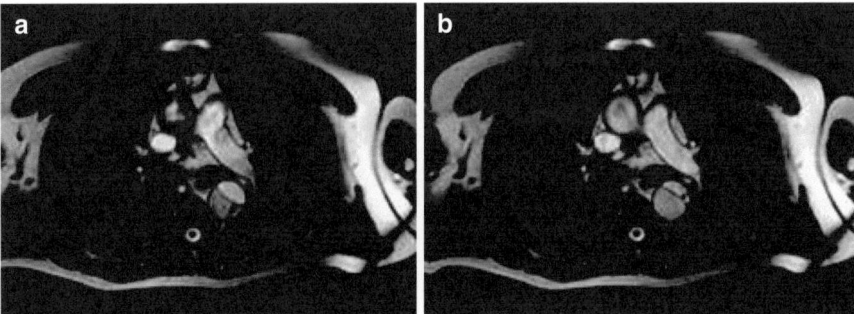

Fig. 17.1 MRI examination. Cine-MRI sequences. Aortic dissection with characteristic flagging of the mid-intimal flap consensual with cardiac pulsation. The presence of vascular flows (jets) through the fixations of the intimal flap is indicative of supply of the false lumen. (**a**) Inlet breach; (**b**) Exit breach

Table 17.2 Elements for identification of true and false lumen

True lumen	False lumen
• Generally smaller than the false lumen • Surrounded by wall calcifications (if present) • In continuity with the non-dissected portion of the aorta • Generally gives rise to celiac trunk, superior mesenteric artery, and right renal artery	• Less opacification after contrast media administration for delayed enhancement or chronic thrombosis • Beak sing: acute angle with the intimal flap • Spider's web sign: shoots of endoluminal collagen fibers • Generally occupies the outer curve of the aortic arch in type A DAs • Usually originates in the left renal artery

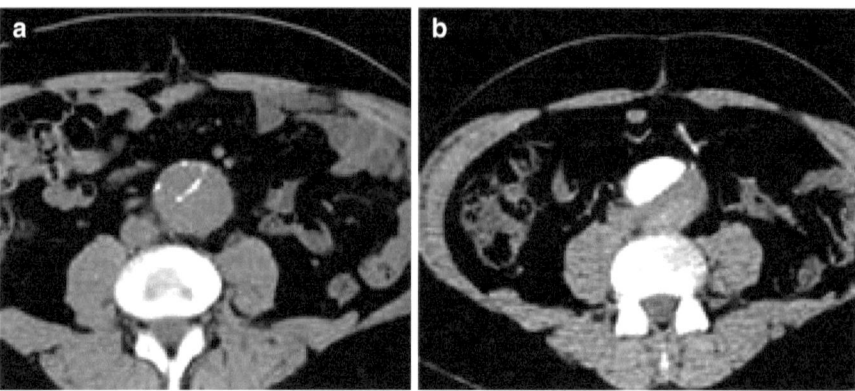

Fig. 17.2 CT examination. (**a**) Pre-contrastografic phase, the true lumen presents smaller size and is surrounded by intimal calcifications; (**b**) Post-contrastografic arterial phase, the false lumen exhibits delayed opacification

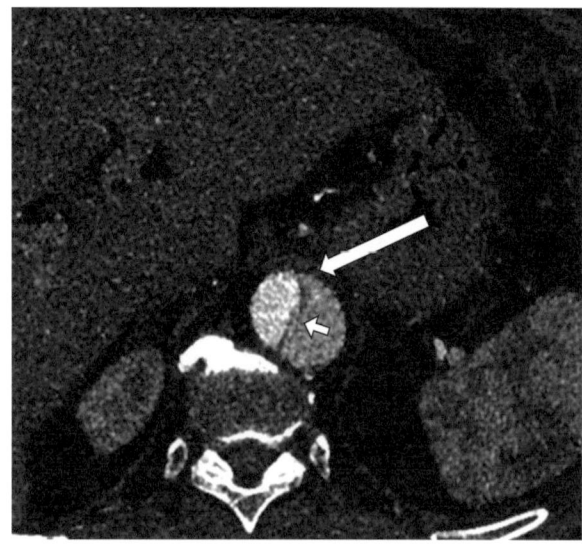

Fig. 17.3 CT examination. The "beak sign" is the acute angle between the intimal flap and the aortic circumference delineating the false lumen (long arrow). The false lumen presents larger dimensions with a characteristic slowed contrast enhancement. "Spider web" sign is indicated by the short arrow

Imaging Techniques

Transthoracic and Transesophageal Echocardiography

The diagnosis of AD with transthoracic echocardiography (ETT) is based on the recognition of the intimal flap separating two aortic lumens. Transesophageal echocardiography (ETE) compared to ETT shows a higher diagnostic accuracy in the study of the entire descending thoracic aorta, since ETT has the ability to detect a distal dissection of the thoracic aorta in only 70% of patients [4]. ETE allows good visualization of the thoracic aorta, especially the ascending tract, the valvular plane and the origin of the coronary arteries. It can be used at the bedside, in the hemodynamically unstable patients, during surgery and in post-surgical monitoring.

The intimal flap is recognized as a linear plus image within the vessel lumen. The size of the true and false lumen depends on the number of communication tears between the two lumens and the time of the dissection [5]. The true lumen is usually smaller than the false lumen and is characterized by systolic expansion with diastolic compliance, as the mid-intimal flap moves in systole toward the false lumen; in contrast, the false lumen is characterized by diastolic expansion with systolic compliance, as the mid-intimal flap moves in diastole toward the true lumen. Color Doppler allows detection of the smallest intimal lesions as flow passes through the intima discontinuity and allows the visualization of entry and re-entry tears between the two lumens and thrombus formation in the false lumen.

ETE, with the use of color Doppler, allows the precise measurement of the size of the tear. In addition, using color Doppler it is possible to document the velocity of anterograde and retrograde flow, while using pulsed or continuous wave Doppler it is possible to estimate the pressure gradients between true and false lumen [6]. For example, a retrograde AD is identified by a lack of flow, reduced or reversed in the false lumen. In case of reduced flow in the false lumen, slow flows known as "smoke effect" can be recorded, which can be attributed to thrombosis in the false lumen. Conversely, the presence of vascular flows in the false lumen is indicative of its reperfusion. The main limitations of this method lie in the impossibility of assessing thoracoabdominal complications and of evaluating the correct measurements of aortic diameters, which are necessary in the pre-surgical evaluation in case of repair by endovascular prostheses [7].

Computed Tomography

CTA, being a rapid and non-invasive imaging technique, constitutes the gold standard for the diagnosis of AD, intramural hematoma and penetrating ulcer, especially in emergency cases [8]. CT provides an accurate three-dimensional comprehensive assessment of the aorta and more generally of the arterial tree, epiaortic vessels, iliac arteries and vasculature of the abdominal organs, useful for preoperative surgical evaluation. CTA has a sensitivity ranging from 96% to 100% and a specificity ranging from 96% to 100% for the diagnosis of acute AD [9].

The correct report of the CTA must indicate the extension of the aorta involved for the right planning of the type of intervention. In particular, if the dissection involves the ascending aorta (Stanford A), this is a surgical emergency and open surgery is planned, while in type B AD complicated by signs of low organ perfusion or disease progression, implantation of an endoprosthesis (TEVAR) is required; on the contrary, in uncomplicated and more distal type B AD, conservative medical treatment is preferred [10].

The CTA protocol for the study of AD consists of in a triphasic angiographic study with a pre-contrastographic phase, an arterial phase, and a venous phase (at approximately 60–120 s after contrast administration). The baseline study is critical for the identification of intramural hematoma, hemothorax, or hemopericardium (Fig. 17.4). The scan volume includes the entire thorax, abdomen, and pelvis in order to visualize the entire aorta and the origin of the vessels and possible organ ischemia, e.g., intestinal or renal [10].

The use of ECG gating allows a considerable improvement in image quality by precisely differentiating motion artifacts in the ascending aorta (pseudoflap) from true aortic dissection [11]. The ECG gating technique can be retrospective, with acquisition during the whole cardiac cycle, or prospective, with acquisition during a specific phase of the cardiac cycle, usually diastole.

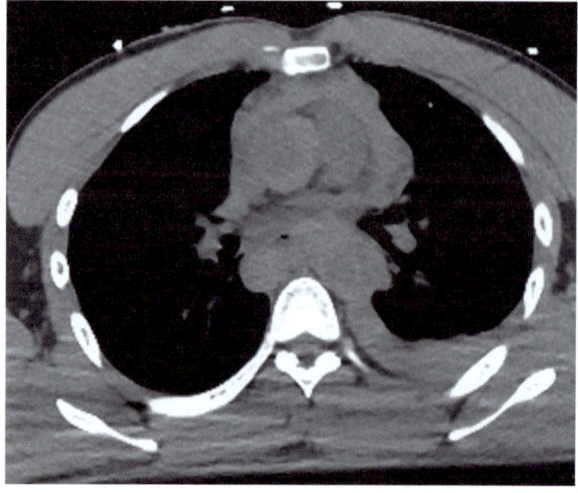

Fig. 17.4 CT examination. Extensive hematoma with circumferential distribution in the ascending aorta. Hemopericardium and hemothorax are associated

Retrospective acquisition allows reduction of artifacts due to cardiac arrhythmias or respiratory movements, but the radiation dose is higher compared to prospective acquisition [12].

In recent years, the introduction of Dual Source (DS) CT scanners, which acquire images using two separate tubes [13], has allowed full-body scans with submillimeter resolution in a few milliseconds. The diagnostic advantages are two: the reduction of pulse artifacts in the ascending aorta (possible even without gating) and the identification of even submillimeter fenestrations, which can influence the decision on the choice of endoprosthesis [10, 14].

The DSCT can allow to reduce the iodinated contrast dose and the radiation dose. Indeed, the use of low kVp (70–80 kVp) results in greater vessel attenuation, and the volume of contrast media can be significantly reduced while maintaining the same image quality. Reducing the contrast dose limits the risk of nephrotoxicity, especially in patients with chronic renal insufficiency or undergoing multiple contrastographic procedures [15].

A new technique introduced by modern CT scanners is time-resolved (or dynamic-4D) CT, in which an anatomical volume of interest can be studied in real time by moving the patient back and forth along the CT gantry for a certain distance (fixed up to 48 cm in Dual Source CT scanners) in order to assess dynamic changes in contrastographic flow [16]. The blood flow can be studied during the cardiac cycle in different phases, producing an angiographic rendering. Time-resolved CTA of the whole aorta is possible with a low radiation dose (<30 mSv), comparable to the radiation dose of standard triphasic protocols, and adds relevant diagnostic information with therapeutic consequences in patients with acute AD [17]. In particular, compared to the traditional triphasic protocol, time-resolved CTA allows to evaluate the different opacification time between true and false lumen, the degree of oscillation of the mid-intimal flap, the perfusion delay of the arteries originating from the false lumen, the quantitative assessment of renal artery perfusion and the dynamic occlusion of aortic arterial branches [17].

Magnetic Resonance Imaging

MRI is considered a very accurate technique for the diagnosis of AD, with sensitivity and specificity of 98% [2]. Similar to CT, it allows a comprehensive study of the aorta, assessing the extent of pathology and showing the distal ascending aorta and aortic arch more precisely than with ETE. The localization of the entrance and re-entry tear is almost as accurate as with ETE and the sensitivity for both is close to 90%. MRI is also very useful in detecting the presence of pericardial effusion, aortic valve insufficiency, or epiaortic vessel dissection In addition, the origin of the proximal coronary arteries and their involvement in the dissection can be visualized [18].

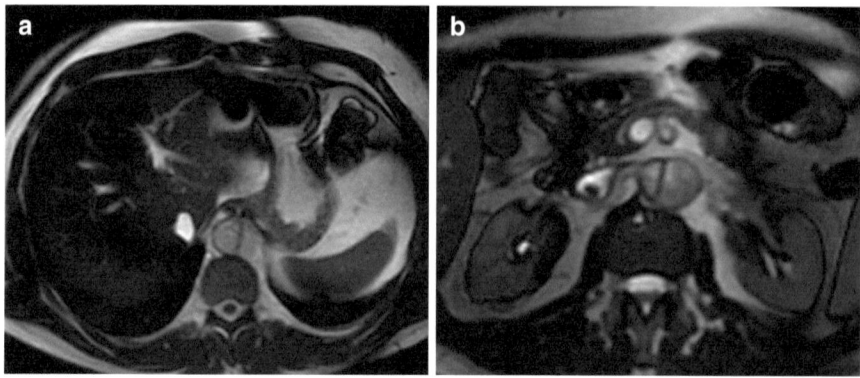

Fig. 17.5 MRI examination. Aortic dissection with emergence of the celiac trunk and right renal artery from the true lumen (**a** and **b**)

After performing localization sequences, "black blood" and "bright blood" vascular sequences are acquired, followed by post-gadolinium gradient echo (GRE) acquisitions (Fig. 17.5). The identification of the intimal flap in the aortic lumen constitutes the main sign of AD, usually well recognized on spin echo (black blood) sequences. The true lumen shows low signal, whereas the false lumen shows high signal intensity, indicative of turbulent flow, thrombosis, or the presence of a slow flow [19].

To quantify the flow in the true lumen and false lumen, cine-SSFP sequences can also be acquired, which are also useful for a better definition of the intimal flap, particularly at the level of the aortic bulb. The motion of the mid-intimal flap is characteristically consensual to the cardiac pulsation. In addition, dynamic sequences and "phase-contrast" sequences can also be acquired. Dynamic sequences, with high temporal resolution (time-resolved), are useful in the study of parenchymal organ perfusion for subsequent therapeutic-surgical planning. Phase-contrast sequences allow to identify the direction of flow in the false lumen and to determine a possible aortic valve regurgitation [20].

Post-contrast GRE sequences highlight the different contrastographic dynamics between the two lumens, with characteristic delayed filling of the false lumen compared to the true one.

Three-dimensional post-contrast sequences (CE-MRA 3D) allow accurate evaluation of the aorta and the branches originating from it (Fig. 17.6). Although MRI have demonstrated high diagnostic accuracy for the diagnosis of acute aortic pathology, it is rarely in clinical practice due to the long time needed for the examination especially in most unstable patients. In contrast, MRI represents a widely used method in the follow-up of aortic syndromes, particularly in young adults. In patients treated with endoprostheses, image quality and diagnostic power may be partially degraded by artifacts generated by the metal mesh [21].

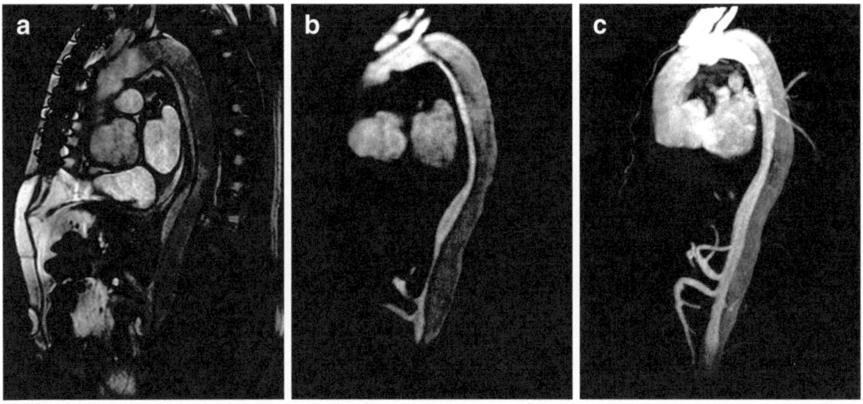

17 Aortic Dissection: Imaging and Elements of Endovascular Pretreatment Evaluation

Fig. 17.6 MRI examination. (**a**) Cine-RM sequence. (**b**) Angio-RM sequence. (**c**) MIP image. The intimal flap is visible as a dark line between the true and false lumen: differences of blood flow velocity show higher signal intensity (white) in the true lumen and lower signal intensity (gray) in the false lumen. Origin of the celiac and superior mesenteric artery from the true lumen

Aortography

The aortography diagnosis of AD is based on "direct" signs, such as visualization of the intimal flap (a minus, often mobile, linear image) or recognition of two separate lumens. "Indirect" signs are represented by the irregularities of the aortic lumen contours, abnormalities of the epiaortic branches, thickening of the aortic wall or aortic valve insufficiency. This technique is no longer used in the diagnostic process of AD, except during coronarography or endovascular surgery, where the diagnosis may be incidental [22].

Chest X-Ray

CXR is commonly requested in patients with acute chest pain and a new-onset mediastinal widening on radiograph may be suspicious for AD. However, this finding has a low specificity, as many other conditions can cause apparent mediastinal widening. Other radiographic findings that may suggest AD are:

- "Double aortic profile" sign: diffuse enlargement of the aorta with poor definition or irregularity of the aortic contour;
- "Calcium sign": separation of the calcific intima from the outer aortic margin by more than 10 mm (Fig. 17.7);
- Pleural effusion: common in descending aortic dissections, usually on the left side;

Fig. 17.7 CXR with diffuse enlargement of the aorta with poor definition and irregularity of the aortic contour, separation of the calcific intima from the outer aortic margin by more than 10 mm and tracheal deviation to the right

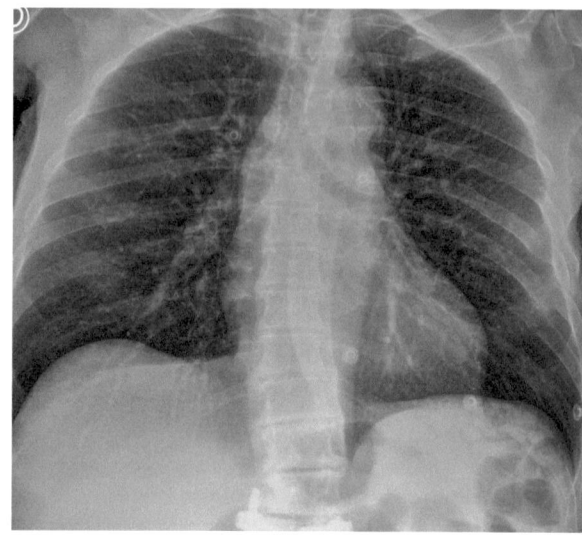

- Tracheal deviation to the right;
- Increased cardiac shadowing in cases of pericardial effusion

CXR lacks in sensitivity and specificity, so the diagnosis may be delayed in up to 40% of patients [23]. For example, the presence of aortic dilatation (left superior mediastinal first arch) is a sign with low sensitivity because AD often does not result in radiographically visible dilatation of the aorta, and with a low specificity because it may be a sign of a chronic aneurysm. The European Society of Cardiology AD-guidelines include CXR among the diagnostic tests in patients with a low-pretest probability of AD [10]. Indeed, CXR due to its minimal sensitivity is not included in fast-track diagnostic pathways in patients with a high pre-test probability because, approximately 12–20% of AD, are undetectable by CXR alone and, therefore, a negative chest radiographic examination does not rule out AD [23].

References

1. Rogers AM, Hermann LK, Booher AM, et al. Sensitivity of the aortic dissection detection risk score, a novel guideline-based tool for identification of acute aortic dissection at initial presentation: results from the international registry of acute aortic dissection. Circulation. 2011;123:2213–8.
2. Nienaber CA, von Kodolitsch Y, Nicolas V, et al. The diagnosis of thoracic aortic dissection by non-invasive imaging procedures. N Engl J Med. 1993;328:1–9.
3. Erbel R, Alfonso F, Boileau C, et al. Diagnosis and management of aortic dissection. Eur Heart J. 2001;2:1642–81.
4. Iliceto S, Ettorre G, Francioso G, et al. Diagnosis of aneurysm of the thoracic aorta. Comparison between two non-invasive techniques: two-dimensional echocardiography and computed tomography. Eur Heart J. 1984;5:545–55.

5. Erbel R, Engberding R, Daniel W, et al. Echocardiography in diagnosis of aortic dissection. Lancet. 1989;1:457–61.
6. Mohr-Kahaly S, Erbel R, Rennollet H, et al. Ambulatory follow-up of aortic dissection by transesophageal two-dimensional and color-coded Doppler echocardiography. Circulation. 1989;80:24–33.
7. Erbel R, Oelert H, Meyer J, et al. Effect of medical and surgical therapy on aortic dissection evaluated by transesophageal echocardiography. Implications for prognosis and therapy. The European Cooperative Study Group on Echocardiography. Circulation. 1993;87:1604–521.
8. Duran ES, Ahmad F, Elshikh M, et al. Computed tomography imaging findings of acute aortic pathologies. Cureus. 2019;11(8):e5534.
9. Sebastià C, Pallisa E, Quiroga S, et al. Aortic dissection: diagnosis and follow-up with helical CT. Radiographics. 1999;19(1):45–60; quiz 149–50.
10. Erbel R, Aboyans V, Boileau C, et al. ESC Committee for Practice Guidelines. 2014 ESC guidelines on the diagnosis and treatment of aortic diseases: document covering acute and chronic aortic diseases of the thoracic and abdominal aorta of the adult. The Task Force for the Diagnosis and Treatment of Aortic Diseases of the European Society of Cardiology (ESC). Eur Heart J. 2014;35(41):2873–926. Erratum in: Eur Heart J 2015; 36(41):2779.
11. Lumia D, Carrafiello G, Laganà D, et al. Diagnosis with ECG-gated MDCT of floating thrombus in aortic arch in a patient with type-A dissection. Vasc Health Risk Manag. 2008;4(3):735–9.
12. Schernthaner RE, Stadler A, Beitzke D, et al. Dose modulated retrospective ECG-gated versus non-gated 64-row CT angiography of the aorta at the same radiation dose: comparison of motion artifacts, diagnostic confidence and signal-to-noise-ratios. Eur J Radiol. 2012;81(4):e585–90.
13. Sawada Y, Shimohira M, Nakagawa M, et al. Advanced monoenergetic reconstruction technique for dual-energy computed tomography to evaluate endoleaks after endovascular stent-graft placement. Abdom Radiol (NY). 2020;45(8):2569–75.
14. Schicchi N, Fogante M, Pirani PE, et al. Third generation dual source CT with ultra-high pitch protocol for TAVI planning and coronary tree assessment: feasibility, image quality and diagnostic performance. Eur J Radiol. 2020;122:108749.
15. Mahoney R, Pavitt CW, Gordon D, et al. Clinical validation of dual-source dual-energy computed tomography (DECT) for coronary and valve imaging in patients undergoing transcatheter aortic valve implantation (TAVI). Clin Radiol. 2014;69(8):786–94.
16. Horinouchi H, Sofue K, Nishii T, et al. CT angiography with 15 mL contrast material injection on time-resolved imaging for endovascular abdominal aortic aneurysm repair. Eur J Radiol. 2020;126:108861.
17. Meinel FG, Nikolaou K, Weidenhagen R, et al. Time-resolved CT angiography in aortic dissection. Eur J Radiol. 2012;81(11):3254–61.
18. Wagner S, Auffermann W, Buser P, et al. Diagnostic accuracy and estimation of the severity of valvular regurgitation from the signal void on cine magnetic resonance images. Am Heart J. 1989;118:760–7.
19. Sakamoto I, Sueyoshi E, Uetani M. MR imaging of the aorta. Radiol Clin North Am. 2007;45:485–97, viii.
20. Sherrah AG, Grieve SM, Jeremy RW, et al. MRI in chronic aortic dissection: a systematic review and future directions. Front Cardiovasc Med. 2015;2:5.
21. Goldstein SA, Evangelista A, Abbara S, et al. Multimodality imaging of diseases of the thoracic aorta in adults: from the American Society of Echocardiography and the European Association of Cardiovascular Imaging: endorsed by the Society of Cardiovascular Computed Tomography and Society for Cardiovascular Magnetic Resonance. J Am Soc Echocardiogr. 2015;28(2):119–82.
22. Baliga RR, Nienaber CA, Bossone E, et al. The role of imaging in aortic dissection and related syndromes. JACC Cardiovasc Imaging. 2014;7(4):406–24.
23. McMahon MA, Squirrell CA. Multidetector CT of aortic dissection: a pictorial review. Radiographics. 2010;30(2):445–60.

Reporting Checklist: Acute Aortic Syndromes 18

Filippo Vaccher

Intramural Hematoma (IMH)

- Proximal involvement: Stanford A vs. B
- Length of aortic hematoma
- Splanchnic vessel involvement
- Maximum hematoma thickness
- Maximum aortic diameter
- Intramural effusion (intramural blood pool, ulcer-like projections, signs of dissection)
- Periaortic alterations (hematoma, adipose tissue inhomogeneity, pericardial effusion, pleural effusion)
- Information for operative planning (vascular anatomical variants, proximal and distal landing zones, vascular accesses routes)

Penetrating Ulcer (PAU)

- Localization/multifocal
- PAU description:
    depth
    longitudinal extent
    vascular collar
    maximum aortic diameter
    partial thrombosis.

F. Vaccher (✉)
Institute of Radiology, Department of Medical and Surgical Specialties, Radiological Sciences, and Public Health, University of Brescia, Brescia, Italy

Radiology Unit 1, ASST Spedali Civili di Brescia, Brescia, Italy

© The Author(s), under exclusive license to Springer Nature Switzerland AG 2024
I. Carbone et al. (eds.), *Imaging of the Aorta*,
https://doi.org/10.1007/978-3-031-52527-8_18

- Complication signs (IMH, dissection, periaortic hematoma)
- Extra-aortic findings (pleural/pericardial effusion)

Traumatic Aortic Injury (TAITAR?)

- Localization and extent of aortic damage
- Degree of aortic damage (type I–IV)
- Extra-luminal Active contrast medium leakage or signs of impending rupture (hemopericardium, hemothorax)
- Associated traumatic injuries (vertebral, cranial, parenchymatous organ contusions, fractures, actively bleeding hematomas)
- Information for operative planning (anatomical variants, aortic diameter, proximal and distal landing zones, in particular distance from left subclavian artery origin, vascular accesses routes)

Aortic Dissection (AD)

- Proximal involvement: Stanford A vs. B
- Intimal flap extension
- True/false lumen relationship (true lumen compression, delayed flow, false lumen thrombosis)
- Involvement of aortic root structures (valvular plane, coronary ostia, hemopericardium)
- Involvement of splanchnic vessels:
    origin from true/false lumen
    static/dynamic obstruction
- End organ ischemia: renal perfusion/intestinal ischemia/organ infarcts
- Identifiable intimal re-entry tears (number, location, extent)
- Information for operative planning:
    possible anatomical (bovine trunk, accessory renal arteries, mesenteric/tripod artery variant, left retro-aortic renal vein) or post-surgical (aorto-coronary bypass or from internal mammary) anatomical variants;
    proximal landing zone (diameter, length, distance from epiaortic vessels ostia, calcifications, tortuosity)
    vascular accesses at the iliac and subclavian arteries (diameter, tortuosity, calcifications, atheromasic disease and chronic occlusions)
    epiaortic vessels (dominant vertebral artery, significant carotid or vertebral atheromasia)

Part VI

Inflammatory Diseases of the Aorta

Imaging Methods: General Principles

19

Filippo Vaccher, Davide Farina, Emanuela Algeri, and Marco Ravanelli

Different imaging methods can be used to evaluate patients with suspected aortic infections. The objectives can be summarized as follows:

(a) To identify signs of vessel wall inflammation—acute or chronic (edema, fibrosis); these elements can be useful in supporting or suggesting the clinical diagnosis, quantifying disease extension and possibly giving information on treatment response/presence of recurrence.
(b) To provide elements useful in formulating a differential diagnosis between the various forms; it is of proven value, for example, in the distinction between aortitis and other causes of vessel degeneration, or between infectious and non-infectious aortitis.
(c) To monitor over time the structural changes in the great vessels (e.g., stenosis, aneurysmal degeneration) and identify late onset complications (e.g., intramural hematoma, dissection, ulceration, rupture or thrombosis).

F. Vaccher · M. Ravanelli
Institute of Radiology, Department of Medical and Surgical Specialties, Radiological Sciences, and Public Health, University of Brescia, Brescia, Italy
e-mail: marco.ravanelli@unibs.it

D. Farina (✉)
Institute of Radiology, Department of Medical and Surgical Specialties, Radiological Sciences, and Public Health, University of Brescia, Brescia, Italy

Radiology Unit 2, ASST Spedali Civili di Brescia, Brescia, Italy
e-mail: davide.farina@unibs.it

E. Algeri
Service de Radiologie et Imagerie Cardiovasculaire, Hôpital Cardiologique, Centre Hospitalier Régional et Universitaire de Lille, Lille Cedex, France

© The Author(s), under exclusive license to Springer Nature Switzerland AG 2024
I. Carbone et al. (eds.), *Imaging of the Aorta*,
https://doi.org/10.1007/978-3-031-52527-8_19

Echocardiography

According to a recent meta-analysis, in patients with large vessel vasculitis, echocardiography has a sensitivity of 77% and specificity of 96% in defining the final diagnosis [1]. Echographic semeiotics consists of three basic elements:

- Parietal edema, visible as a hypoechoic perivascular sleeve, correlated with localization of active inflammation and, when regression is observed during follow-up, with response to therapy [2]; it is described as "halo sign" in Giant Cell Arteritis and as "macaroni sign" in Takayasu (see below).
- Parietal thickening (due to increased medio-intimal thickness).
- Aneurysmal dilatation and chronic vascular degeneration.

CT-Angiography (CTA)

CTA is the most commonly used morphological imaging method, extremely effective for its wide availability and rapidity of execution, associated with high spatial and temporal resolution. The basic elements of CTA semeiotics are:

- Parietal thickening: to be considered positive if >2–3 mm, concentric.
- Parietal enhancement: highly specific "double ring sign" in the equilibrium phase, with concentric enhancement of adventitial/medial layers and weak intimal enhancement, suggestive of edema; it seems to be associated with active disease (Fig. 19.1).
- Perivascular findings: retroperitoneal periaortic adenopathies; periaortic adipose tissue inhomogeneity (fat stranding)/perivascular fibrosis.
- Chronic vascular changes: aneurysmal degeneration, stenosis, occlusion.
- Acute complications: thrombosis, intramural hematoma, dissection, rupture.

Some elements of CT semeiotics allow differentiating parietal thickening caused by aortic inflammatory disease from that related to the presence of IMH (Table 19.1).

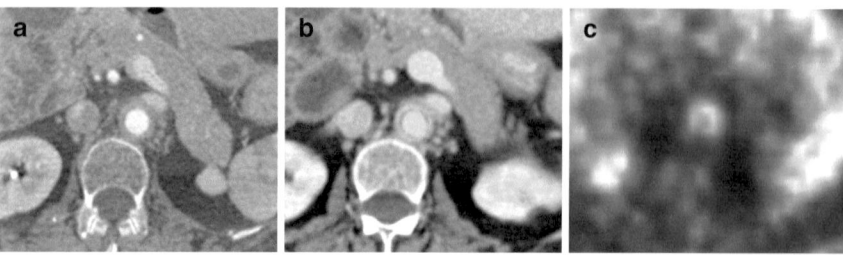

Fig. 19.1 CT angiography (**a**) demonstrates circumferential aortic wall thickening with intense peripheral enhancement at equilibrium phase; intimal hypodensity contributes to determine the double ring sign, suggestive of active disease (**b**). Active inflammation is confirmed by the tracer uptake in PET-CT (**c**)

Table 19.1 Inflammatory disease (ID) vs. intramural hematoma (IMH)

	ID	IMH
Shape	Circumferential	Crescentic, asymmetric
Density (no-contrast CT)	Low (25–30 HU)	High (45–50 HU)
Enhancement	High (75–80 HU)	None

PET-CT

It is a functional imaging modality that assesses the accumulation of 18F-FDG (fluorodeoxyglucose) in various anatomical structures, being that FDG transport across cell membranes is proportional to cellular glucose uptake. Glycolytic activity is increased in tumor cells and in those cells that mediate flogosis, particularly in macrophages and lymphocytes. PET imaging in vasculitis is based, therefore, on the indirect identification (by the presence of 18F-FDG) of inflammatory cells infiltrating the vascular wall and perivascular tissue. Any tracer accumulation is considered pathological at the level of the vessel wall, which is normally devoid of any. The uptake intensity of the liver parenchyma is used as a reference level (uptake considered pathological if equal to or greater than that of the liver parenchyma), although qualitative assessment of the uptake is still considered superior to semiquantitative analyses (because of reported higher specificity) [3]. Data from the literature attribute to PET-CT 80–92% sensitivity and 88–100% specificity in identifying active inflammation in patients with arteritis [4–6].

However, spatial resolution is limited (4–8 mm) and radiant exposure is high, which greatly limits its use, particularly in the long-term follow-up of young patients.

FDG-PET semeiotics consists essentially in the demonstration of tracer uptake, evaluated according to different semiquantitative and dimensionless scales. The most frequently used ones are the SUV or Standardized Uptake Value (ratio between activity detected in a certain region per grams of tissue and activity injected per unit of body weight) and qualitative grading (0 = no activity detected; 1 = activity less than hepatic uptake; 2 = activity equivalent to hepatic uptake; 3 = activity greater than hepatic uptake) [7]. Generally, uptake is greater than or equal to that of homogeneous and extensive liver uptake.

Importantly, uptake can also be observed in atherosclerotic lesions, although in this case it frequently appears focal (spotty pattern) and of low intensity (lower than hepatic uptake). Moreover, atherosclerotic lesions' uptake coincides with the localization of the largest plaques on morphological imaging and is mostly located in the abdominal aorta and iliac-femoral vessels.

MRI

Although it has lower spatial resolution than CTA, MRI plays a key role in the study of aortic inflammatory disease by virtue of its high contrast resolution, which allows superior tissue characterization compared to CTA. This may prove essential not only for the evaluation of inflammatory changes of the aortic wall, but also for the identification of inflammatory lesions of the periaortic tissues and of retroperitoneal fibrosis. In addition, Phase-Contrast and 4D-Flow sequences allow qualitative and quantitative assessment of flows. The main intrinsic limitation of this technique is the poor representation of calcium.

The combination of morphological and angiographic MRI sequences can demonstrate:

- Parietal thickening and edema: in particular, wall hyperintensity in T2 fat-sat sequences is an early sign of disease, which makes the sensitivity of MRI superior than that of CTA (although in any case inferior to PET-CT).
- Parietal enhancement: highlighted by black-blood T1 sequences or by subtraction of pre- and post-contrastographic images.
- Perivascular alterations: in the case of periaortitis, represented by tissue sleeve T1-hypointense and T2-hyperintense, highly enhancing after contrast medium administration; in the case of retroperitoneal fibrosis, instead, the tissue is generally hypointense both in T1 and T2 weighted sequences, although the T2 signal may depend on the stage of the disease.
- Chronic vascular modifications: aneurysmal degeneration, stenosis, occlusion.

References

1. Duftner C, Dejaco C, Sepriano A, et al. Imaging in diagnosis, outcome prediction and monitoring of large vessel vasculitis: a systematic literature review and meta-analysis informing the EULAR recommendations. RMD Open. 2018;4(1):e000612.
2. Gornik HL, Creager MA. Aortitis. Circulation. 2008;117(23):3039–51.
3. Puppo C, Massollo M, Paparo F, et al. Giant cell arteritis: a systematic review of the qualitative and semiquantitative methods to assess vasculitis with 18F-fluorodeoxyglucose positron emission tomography. Biomed Res Int. 2014;2014:574248.
4. Kobayashi Y, Ishii K, Oda K, et al. Aortic wall inflammation due to Takayasu arteritis imaged with 18F-FDG PET coregistered with enhanced CT. J Nucl Med. 2005;46(6):917–22.
5. Walter MA, Melzer RA, Schindler C, et al. The value of [18F]FDG-PET in the diagnosis of large-vessel vasculitis and the assessment of activity and extent of disease. Eur J Nucl Med Mol Imaging. 2005;32(6):674–81.
6. Webb M, Chambers A, AL-Nahhas A, et al. The role of 18F-FDG PET in characterising disease activity in Takayasu arteritis. Eur J Nucl Med Mol Imaging. 2004;31(5):627–34.
7. Bossone E, Pluchinotta FR, Andreas M, et al. Aortitis. Vasc Pharmacol. 2016;80:1–10.

Giant Cell Arteritis, Takayasu Arteritis, Chronic Periaortitis, Infectious Aortitis

20

Filippo Vaccher, Davide Farina, Emanuela Algeri, and Marco Ravanelli

Giant Cell Arteritis (GCA)

GCA is a chronic idiopathic granulomatous vasculitis; it represents the most common form of aortitis (incidence 10-19:100.000), typically observed in patients older than 50 years, with lower predilection for the female sex compared to other vasculitides (in particular Takayasu's arteritis). Classically, a cranial phenotype (temporal a., carotid a., vertebral a. involvement) and one with involvement of the large vessels (LV-GCA) are described. In LV-GCA, in order of frequency, the subclavian arteries (75%), thoracic and abdominal aorta (50%), and iliac and femoral arteries (30–40%) are involved [1].

The most typical symptoms of the cranial form are temporal headache, claudication of the jaw, pain, and swelling of the scalp in the temporal region, and visual disturbances. In LV-GCA claudication of the limbs, vascular murmurs and asymmetry of peripheral pulses may occur.

Systemic signs and symptoms may accompany both forms.

F. Vaccher (✉)
Institute of Radiology, Department of Medical and Surgical Specialties, Radiological Sciences, and Public Health, University of Brescia, Brescia, Italy

Radiology Unit 1, ASST Spedali Civili di Brescia, Brescia, Italy

D. Farina · M. Ravanelli
Institute of Radiology, Department of Medical and Surgical Specialties, Radiological Sciences, and Public Health, University of Brescia, Brescia, Italy

Radiology Unit 2, ASST Spedali Civili di Brescia, Brescia, Italy
e-mail: davide.farina@unibs.it; marco.ravanelli@unibs.it

E. Algeri
Service de Radiologie et Imagerie Cardiovasculaire, Hôpital Cardiologique, Centre Hospitalier Régional et Universitaire de Lille, Lille Cedex, France

© The Author(s), under exclusive license to Springer Nature Switzerland AG 2024
I. Carbone et al. (eds.), *Imaging of the Aorta*,
https://doi.org/10.1007/978-3-031-52527-8_20

LV-GCA produces marked, segmental, and often symmetrical parietal thickening, with similar degree of involvement of those arteries on both sides of the body (e.g., subclavian, temporal, iliac arteries).

Imaging plays a key role in the diagnosis of the disease. Ultrasonography (possibly also used as a guide for biopsy) is critical in cases where signs indicative of cranial involvement predominate. Typically, ultrasonography demonstrates the "halo sign," a finding generated by the thickening of the medio-intimal complex and the presence of a perivascular hypoechogenic layer; the poor compressibility of the thickened wall in the involved arterial segment is also quite characteristic.

Panoramic study with PET-CT, CTA or MRI is indicated in patients with predominant cranial symptoms when the temporal a. biopsy is negative but the clinical probability of disease is intermediate to high, or when the biopsy is positive (to complete staging of the disease) (Fig. 20.1). On the contrary, in patients with prevalent extracranial symptoms, PET-CT, CTA, or MRI study acts as a gatekeeper for the execution of biopsy: if positive, it allows the diagnosis without the need for

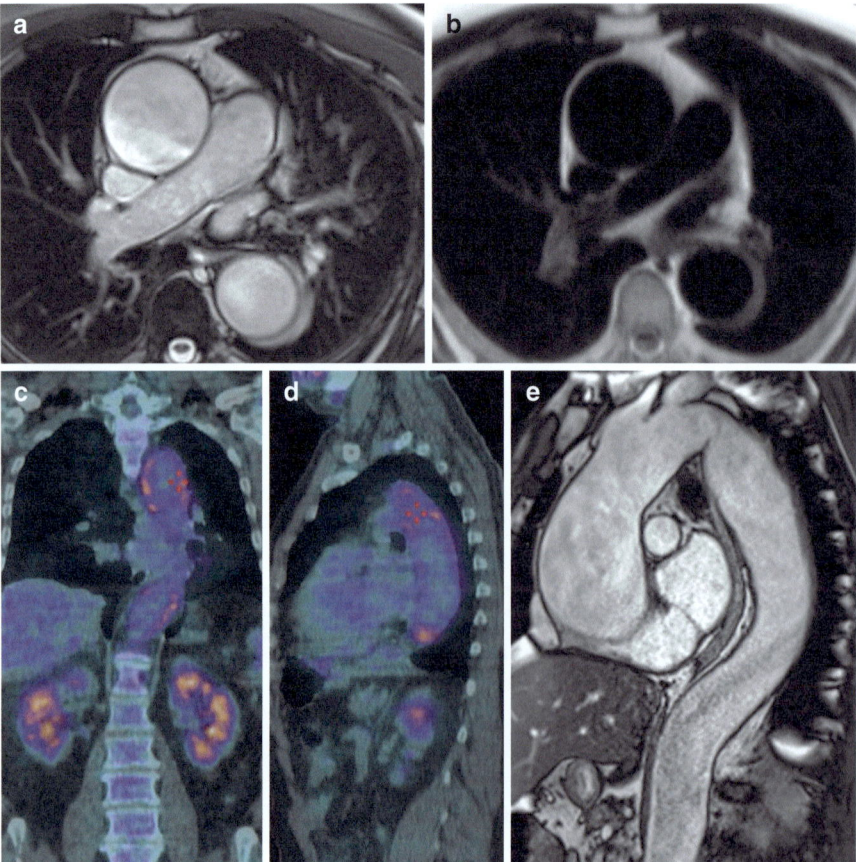

Fig. 20.1 Giant cell arteritis. Aneurysm of the ascending aorta. Extensive parietal thickening of the descending aorta; signal hyperintensity in T2-weighted bright blood sequences (**a**, **e**) and intermediate signal in the T1-weighted black blood sequences (**b**) suggest active disease. The suspicion is confirmed by the tracer uptake demonstrated with PET-CT (**c**, **d**)

biopsy. In this scenario, biopsy is indicated only if panoramic imaging is negative, but the clinical probability is intermediate to high.

Up to now, there is no established consensus on PET-CT, CTA or MRI timing in the follow-up: monitoring is based on clinical assessment and laboratory findings; imaging (in particular PET-CT and MRI) is indicated if necessary to confirm the clinical suspicion of flare-up or to look for new vascular lesions. Importantly, aneurysmal degeneration of the aorta is common in the late stages of the disease: the relative risk of thoracic aortic aneurysm in patients with GCA is 17 times that of the control population, with high mortality due to acute aortic complication [2].

Takayasu's Arteritis

Rare form of vasculitis, much less frequent than GCA (incidence 0.4–2.6/1,000,000), typical of the female sex (M:F 1:6–8) and more commonly diagnosed in the third decade of life (mean age at diagnosis 25–30 years) [3].

Disease course comprises three stages. The early stage, characterized by vague and aspecific symptoms (such as arthralgia and muscular pain, fever, exhaustion, anorexia, and weight loss), which are often the cause of a delayed diagnosis (by 10–15 months on average). In the pulseless phase, macroscopic inflammation of the vascular wall is detectable with pain at the affected sites (carotidodynia, thoracic/retroscapular pain, claudication, and symptoms of organ ischemia); asymmetry of arterial pulses and uncontrolled hypertension may also occur in this phase. The third phase, burn-out phase, is characterized by vascular lesions, such as fibrosis and stenosis, and seldom by aneurysmal degeneration (Fig. 20.2).

Relapses are frequent, observed in 45–90% of patients who achieve remission with glucocorticoids per os, while a self-limiting monophasic course of disease is rare (12–20%) [3].

The most commonly affected vessels are the subclavian arteries/brachiocephalic trunk (90%), the descending aorta (60%), the aortic arch, the common carotid arteries (50%) and, with progressively decreasing frequency, the abdominal aorta, renal,

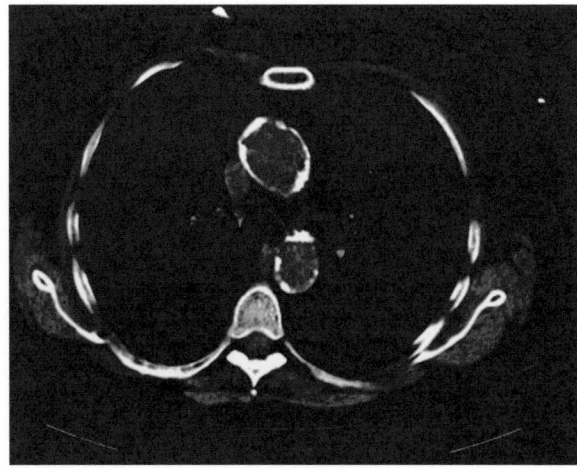

Fig. 20.2 Takayasu arteritis in burn-out phase. Basal CT obtained 20 years after diagnosis demonstrates extensive circumferential parietal calcifications

mesenteric and vertebral arteries. Involvement of coronary arteries (6%) and pulmonary arteries (10%) is less frequent but possible.

MRI should be considered the modality of choice for confirmation of a clinical suspicion, given the characteristics of the population of reference (young women mostly affected). PET-CT, CTA, and ultrasonography are alternative methods to be used in doubtful cases [4].

Regardless of the technique used, the signs that can be looked for are parietal thickening, stenosis, aneurysmal dilatation and parietal calcifications. The parietal thickening is greater in the acute phase, when, however, the vessel luminal diameter is maintained; on the contrary, in the chronic phase, a lower degree of thickening is associated with greater stenosis of the lumen. On ultrasonography, parietal thickening shows bright echogenicity compared with the "halo sign" of GCA and results in an irregular, wavy luminal profile (dubbed macaroni sign).

Moderate/severe segmental stenosis is very frequent (90% of cases); wall irregularities of the affected segments are present in almost all cases.

Aneurysmal degeneration is possible, but rarer than in GCA (20–45%); it generally involves the descending aorta. MRI and CTA may demonstrate parietal ulcers and endoluminal thrombi.

Parietal calcifications, attributed to the burn-out phase and reported after 5 years of disease, are diffuse, extensive, circumferential and continuous, with relative sparing of the ascending aorta; these elements distinguish them from atheromasic calcifications, which instead are generally focal and extremely rare in young women [5]. In addition, the distribution of lesions can be a useful element for the differential diagnosis: in Takayasu's arteritis, the pattern with parietal involvement of long continuous segments prevails (Fig. 20.3); the pattern with "skip lesions" (more similar to what is observed in GCA) is limited to 16% of cases (Fig. 20.4).

Imaging is not indicated in patients in clinical/biochemical remission; it is instead indicated in suspected disease flare, with a complementary role to the

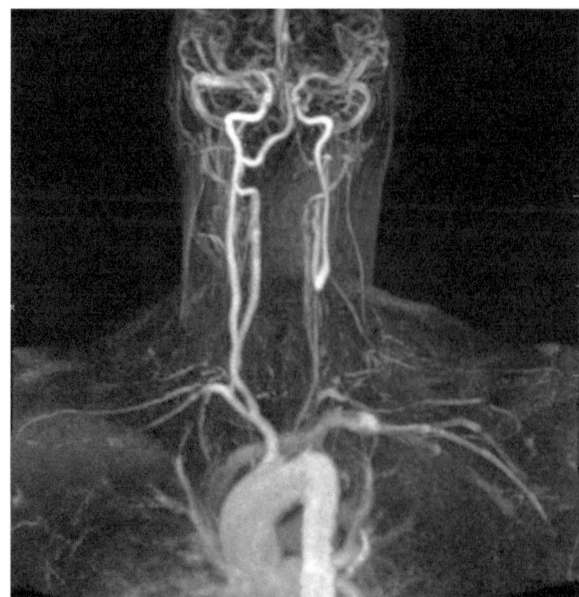

Fig. 20.3 Takayasu arteritis. MIP reconstruction of MR Angiography demonstrates extensive stenosis of the right subclavian artery, substenosis of the left carotid artery, and complete occlusion of the left subclavian artery. Phase-contrast study (not shown) indicated patent distal left subclavian with reversed blood flow into the vertebral ipsilateral artery (subclavian steal syndrome)

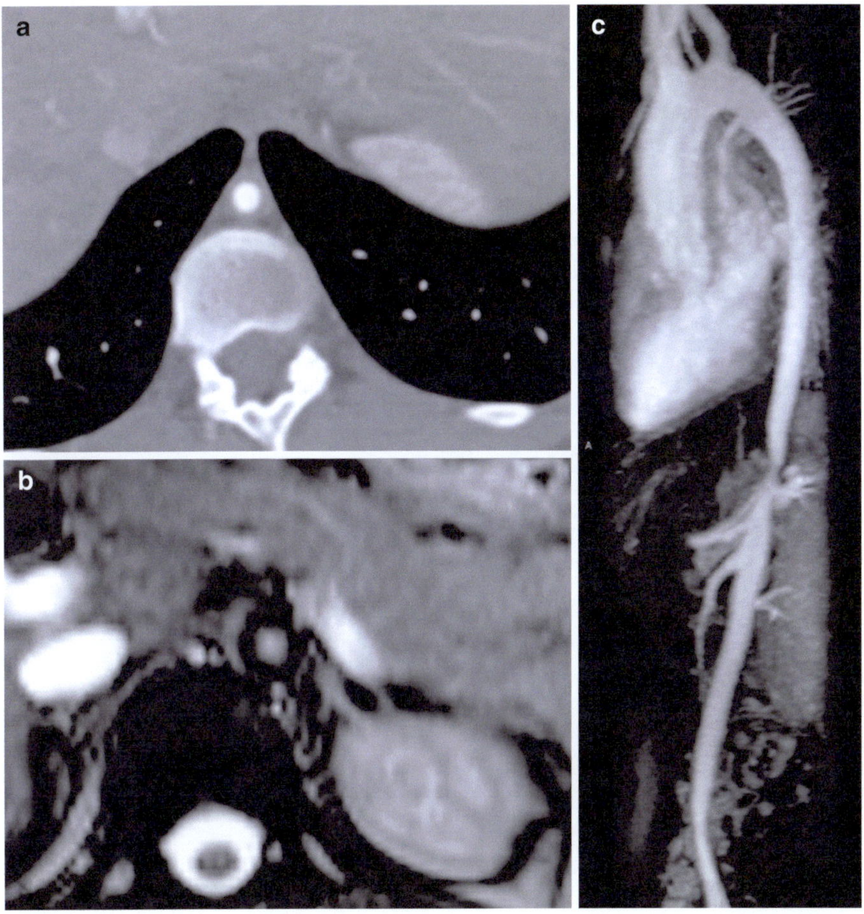

Fig. 20.4 Takayasu arteritis. Stenotic evolution in a patient with focal aortic wall disease. The patient complained lower limb claudication and had refractory hypertension. Both CTA (**a**) and MRI (**b, c**) demonstrated focal aortic stenosis at the thoracoabdominal level. Hypointense T2 signal of the wall indicates fibrosis (smoldering disease)

clinical assessment. PET-CT has a sensitivity of 81% and a specificity of 74% in the diagnosis of disease reactivation; the low specificity is justified by the persistence of tracer uptake in some cases of remission, due to vascular wall smooth muscle remodeling phenomena. MRI seems to have an emerging role for the ability of demonstrating parietal edema as a marker of activity.

Chronic Periaortitis

It is a rare vascular and connective inflammatory disease (incidence 1:200,000) which comprises a spectrum of conditions, the major variant of which is retroperitoneal fibrosis, while the minor ones being IgG4-related disease and inflammatory aneurysm of the abdominal aorta. It is more prevalent in the male sex (M:F 2–3:1) between 40 and 60 years of age. It is idiopathic in most cases (60%); less frequently it might be secondary to peculiar medical therapy (alkaloids, dopaminergics, beta-blockers assumption), complications of trauma settings (retroperitoneal bleeding) or radiotherapy treatment. In 8% of cases, in addition, it consists of a malignant form of desmoplastic fibrosis reactive to neoplasia (lymphoma, retroperitoneal sarcoma, carcinoids, metastases from gastric, ovarian, colon, lung or thyroid cancers) [6].

Retroperitoneal fibrosis consists of an irregular parietal thickening of the aorta (histologically, adventitial and peri-adventitial layers inflammatory infiltration prevails), with linear calcifications on the luminal side and apposition of circumferential periaortic solid tissue on the outer side, the density of which is similar to that of muscle. It usually involves the abdominal aorta, often near the iliac bifurcation (commonly centered at the level of fourth and fifth lumbar vertebra) (Fig. 20.5).

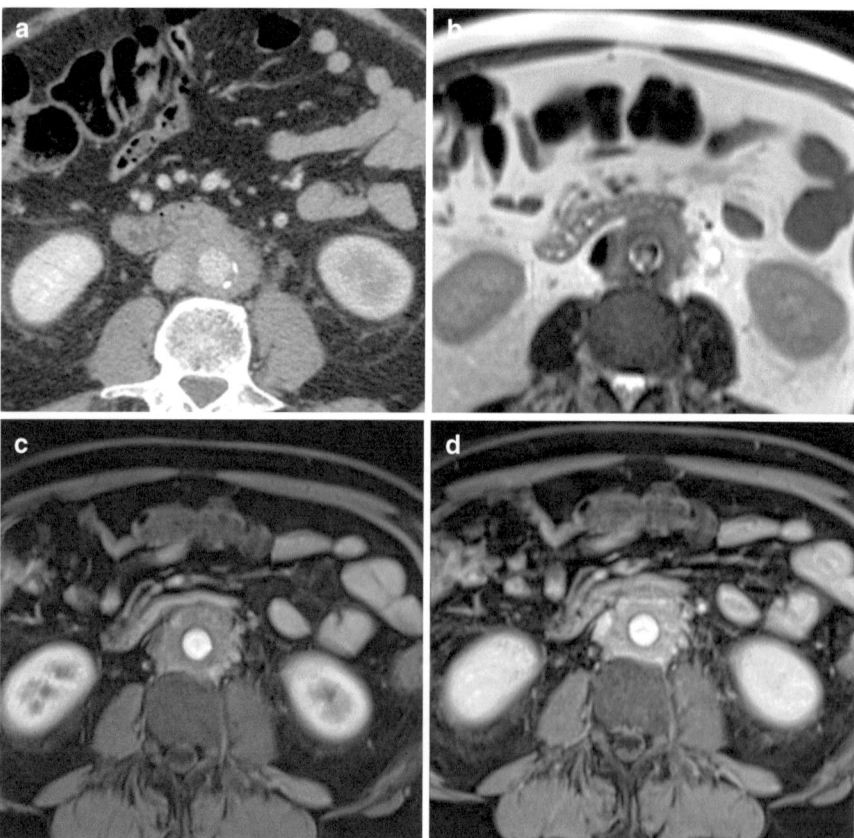

Fig. 20.5 Retroperitoneal fibrosis. Post-contrast CT acquired during delayed phase (**a**) shows homogeneous enhancement of the circumferential parietal thickening. On T2-weighted sequences the signal is mildly hyperintense (**b**). The dynamic study with GE T1 fat-sat sequences shows minimal enhancement in the early phase (**c**), but moderate enhancement in the late phase (**d**). The CT and MRI pattern suggested active disease

The fibrosis begins in proximity to the vessel and extends proximally along its walls and outward to adjacent tissues; it has an infiltrative behavior, with irregular margins, so it respects the arrangement of adjacent anatomical structures, growing between them without macroscopically dislodging them. Rarely, it may have anterior peripancreatic and periduodenal extension and may involve the root of the mesentery [7].

It can cause stenosis of the aorta and its vessels or late aneurysmal degeneration. Frequent complications, often responsible for the symptoms at diagnosis, are due to remodeling of nearby structures: hydroureteronephrosis with post-renal renal failure (due to ureteral obstruction), venous congestion of the lower limbs (due to inferior vena cava compression).

IgG4-related disease is a syndrome characterized by high blood titers of IgG4 antibodies and tissue infiltration of IgG4-positive plasma cells in the involved organs [7, 8]. In this syndrome, chronic periaortitis is associated with multiple organ involvement, such as pancreas (autoimmune pancreatitis), salivary glands (sialadenitis), thyroid (Riedel's fibrous thyroiditis). Biliary tract involvement (sclerosing cholangitis) and mediastinal and pulmonary fibrosis are also described.

Unlikely retroperitoneal fibrosis, IgG4-related disease is characterized by "skip lesions" (multifocal, not continuous), with involvement of the thoracic aorta and aortic arch, increased extension along the origin of splanchnic vessels, and formation of paravertebral masses [9].

Finally, the inflammatory aneurysm of the abdominal aorta is commonly fusiform, distinguished from the classic atherosclerotic aneurysm by the presence of perianeurysmal fibrotic alterations that sometimes spare the posterior wall. The disease location is almost exclusively abdominal; often the affected segment shows advanced and early atherosclerosis, with thick and irregular athero-thrombotic wall plaques. Patients are on average younger and much more frequently symptomatic than those affected by common atherosclerotic abdominal aneurysms [10]. According to some series, inflammatory abdominal aneurysm constitutes 5–25% of all abdominal aortic aneurysms undergoing open repair (OR) [5, 11]. Although the risk of rupture is lower, it is subject to a higher rate of complications from retroperitoneal extension of disease and to a higher intraoperative mortality compared with surgery in common atherosclerotic aneurysms (8% vs. 3%) [12]. In the radiological report it is important to mention any fibrotic adhesions to nearby tissues, in order to aid in the operative planning (retroperitoneal vs. transperitoneal approach) and to report the extent of the disease (infrarenal vs. iuxta/suprarenal).

In chronic periaortitis, CTA and MRI are essential for the initial diagnosis; periaortic tissue may have late and variable enhancement depending on disease activity (20–60 HU enhancement in acute phase; almost null in fibrotic phase). The T1 MRI signal is generally hypointense; the T2 sequence is more informative, showing an intermediate-high signal in the acute phase (due to edema from inflammatory infiltrate) and hypointense in the chronic phase. PET-CT demonstrates uptake correlated with the degree of disease activity, allows to map all sites of disease and guides the choice of bioptic targets. Ultrasonography demonstrates a sleeve of hypoechoic, homogeneous, well-demarcated tissue, displaying irregular contours. The gold standard remains histopathologic evaluation by biopsy, particularly in cases with suspicious radiologic features and little or no response to therapy [6, 7].

CT is the most suitable technique for the evaluation of complications; whereas MRI may require significant increases in examination time. PET-CT is superior in the identification of any associated neoplastic lesions (local, distant primaries or secondary lesions).

As far as the follow-up is concerned, changes in periaortic tissue thickness and in the degree of enhancement, which can both be monitored by CT and MRI, are excellent indicators of disease activity; however, PET-CT is still the most sensitive imaging technique [7].

Infectious Aortitis

Rare clinical entity, but with high mortality (44% despite treatment [13]) and morbidity. It often occurs in patients with pre-existing aortic wall pathology (advanced atherosclerosis, cystic medial necrosis, aneurysms or dissections, prosthetic aortic replacement or EVAR, valve prostheses). In most cases it is caused by bacterial infections (*Salmonella*, enterococci, staphylococci, *S. pneumoniae*); fungal infections affect exclusively immunocompromised patients [13]. Pathogenetic mechanisms may involve colonization of atheromasic plaques by microorganisms present in the bloodstream during septicaemia or sepsis (an event more frequent, for example, following gastrointestinal infections), septic embolization of the vasa vasorum (during endocarditis), direct extension of an external infectious focus to the aortic wall (spondylodiscitis, abscesses, osteomyelitis), direct inoculation as a complication of surgery or trauma [11]. Periprosthetic aortic infection is a rare but feared post-procedural complication (1.3–5% incidence in OR, 1% in EVAR; mortality rates 25–75%) [11, 13].

Radiological warning signs in the postoperative course are the presence of periprosthetic fluid collection beyond 3 months after surgery, increasing extent of postprocedural changes in periaortic tissue, and the presence of air bubbles after the first month following surgery [13].

Infectious aortitis can evolve with the formation of rapidly growing pseudoaneurysms or mycotic saccular aneurysms (Fig. 20.6). Such aneurysms differ from atheromasic ones (usually fusiform in morphology), as they frequently are eccentric and rarely present calcification or athero-thrombotic wall apposition. They are aneurysms at high risk for complications, such as dissection, rupture, and septic embolization.

The clinical symptoms are extremely vague, leaving great importance to imaging findings. CTA is the most suitable imaging technique; the most characteristic findings are asymmetrical crescent-shaped parietal thickening (different from the circumferential one of vasculitis) and aortic wall enhancement. Edema and fat-stranding in the periaortic adipose tissue are frequent; they may evolve to periaortic fluid collection and, in more advanced stages, to abscess formation (e.g., in the psoas) and bone erosion (vertebral bodies, sternal manubrium, or sternoclavicular joints). It is possible to identify air bubbles in the fluid collection or within the thickened walls (this finding is usually poorly depicted on MRI). MRI efficaciously

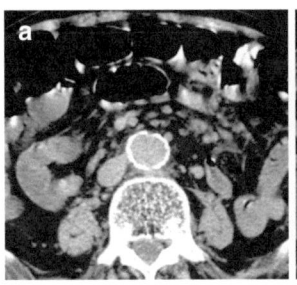 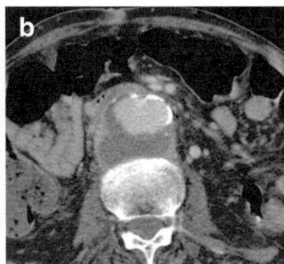 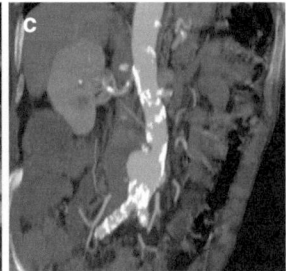

Fig. 20.6 Frail patient admitted for *Salmonella*-associated gastroenteritis. Initial CT findings (**a**) were suggestive of aortitis due to the inhomogeneity of the periaortic adipose tissue, in which several adenopathies can be identified. The CT scan performed 40 days later due to the onset of low back pain (**b, c**) showed development of an inflammatory pseudoaneurysm

demonstrates vascular and perivascular changes; PET may be conclusive in doubtful cases, demonstrating avid inflammatory tracer uptake. At times, some features detectable on imaging may even suggest the etiologic agent. *Salmonella* aortitis has a preferential abdominal localization, with frequent formation of mycotic saccular aneurysms. A history of previous gastrointestinal infection is common. In tubercular aortitis, the involvement is more frequently depicted in the descending aorta or at the aortic arch, with formation of pseudoaneurysm with multilobular contour. Aortic colonization often occurs due to direct extension from pulmonary lesions, lymph nodes, or bone tubercular lesions (lung cavitated lesions, local lymphadenitis, infected pleural effusion, and empyema). In syphilitic aortitis, instead, the ascending aorta (with associated valvular insufficiency) and the aortic arch (where multiple sacciform aneurysms form) are frequently involved; chronic inflammation results in extensive parietal calcification (tree-bark appearance).

In periprosthetic infectious aortitides, it should be remembered that MRI is limited by artifacts created by the metal of the prosthesis. Even with PET-CT examination the diagnostic accuracy can be limited by false positive results, as a consequence of chronic inflammation of the native aortic wall (in EVARs) or of the residual aneurysmal cavity (in ORs), which result in a moderate and diffuse uptake of tracer, especially in the first 3 months after surgery.

In the suspicion of an associated valvular endocarditis, the imaging of choice is transesophageal echocardiography; however, CT scan acquired with cardio-synchronized protocols may allow a more panoramic assessment of the aortic root.

References

1. Schmidt WA, Blockmans D. Investigations in systemic vasculitis—the role of imaging. Best Pract Res Clin Rheumatol. 2018;32(1):63–82.
2. Evans JM, O'Fallon WM, Hunder GG. Increased incidence of aortic aneurysm and dissection in giant cell (temporal) arteritis. A population-based study. Ann Intern Med. 1995;122(7):502–7.
3. Cronenwett JL, Johnston KW, Rutherford RB, editors. Rutherford's vascular surgery. 6th ed. Philadelphia, PA: Elsevier/Saunders; 2005.

4. Dejaco C, Ramiro S, Duftner C, et al. EULAR recommendations for the use of imaging in large vessel vasculitis in clinical practice. Ann Rheum Dis. 2018;77(5):636–43.
5. Restrepo CS, Ocazionez D, Suri R, et al. Aortitis: imaging spectrum of the infectious and inflammatory conditions of the aorta. Radiographics. 2011;31(2):435–51.
6. Cronin CG, Lohan DG, Blake MA, et al. Retroperitoneal fibrosis: a review of clinical features and imaging findings. Am J Roentgenol. 2008;191(2):423–31.
7. Caiafa RO, Vinuesa AS, Izquierdo RS, et al. Retroperitoneal fibrosis: role of imaging in diagnosis and follow-up. Radiographics. 2013;33(2):535–52.
8. Ozawa M, Fujinaga Y, Asano J, et al. Clinical features of IgG4-related periaortitis/periarteritis based on the analysis of 179 patients with IgG4-related disease: a case-control study. Arthritis Res Ther. 2017;19:223.
9. Inoue D, Zen Y, Abo H, et al. Immunoglobulin G4-related periaortitis and periarteritis: CT findings in 17 patients. Radiology. 2011;261(2):625–33.
10. Murphy DJ, Keraliya AR, Agrawal MD, et al. Cross-sectional imaging of aortic infections. Insights Imaging. 2016;7(6):801–18.
11. Hellmann DB, Grand DJ, Freischlag JA. Inflammatory abdominal aortic aneurysm. JAMA. 2007;297(4):395–400. https://doi.org/10.1001/jama.297.4.395. PMID: 17244836.
12. Katabathina VS, Restrepo CS. Infectious and noninfectious aortitis: cross-sectional imaging findings. Semin Ultrasound CT MRI. 2012;33(3):207–21.
13. Poredos P. Inflammatory aortic aneurysm. An article from the E-Journa l of the ESC Council for Cardiology Practice. 2008;7:10–18

21. Reporting Checklist: Inflammatory Diseases of the Aorta

Filippo Vaccher, Davide Farina, Emanuela Algeri, and Marco Ravanelli

- Vessel involvement (indicate the site):
  - large vessels
  - medium vessels
  - both
- Type of involvement:
  - segmental/continuous
  - symmetrical/non-symmetrical
- Status of vessel wall:
  - normal
  - thickened (cut-off 0.6 mm): homogenous/irregular/asymmetrical crescent-shaped
  - presence/absence of calcifications
- Contrast enhancement of vessel wall:
  - absent
  - present (describe the pattern): transmural, layered, delayed

- Signs of infection:
  - air bubbles within vessel wall
- Signs of complications:
  - peri-aortic fat stranding
  - peri-vascular fluid collection
  - aneurysmatic evolution
  - luminal stenosis or vessel occlusion
  - abscess formation (infectious aortitis)

Part VII

Congenital Anomalies of the Thoracic Aorta: An Overview

Aortic Dilatation and Aortopathies in Congenital Heart Disease

22

Paolo Ciancarella, Veronica Bordonaro, and Aurelio Secinaro

Bicuspid Aortic Valve Related Aortopathy

Bicuspid aortic valve (BAV) is the most common congenital cardiovascular disease, with a prevalence of 1–2% in the general population and a male–female ratio 2:1 [1]. It may be associated with other congenital heart diseases such as aortic coarctation, ductus arteriosus patency, subvalvular or supravalvular aortic stenosis/Williams syndrome, interventricular septal defect, and Shone's complex.

There are several morphological classifications based on the presence of fusion raphe, commissures position and valve cups symmetry; the most common is the Sievers classification [2]: in more than 70% of cases, BAV results from fusion of the coronary cusps (type 1 R-L), in 15–20% of cases there is a right/non-coronary cusps fusion (type 1 R-N), while the remaining 5% is a left/non-coronary fusion (type 1 L-N). The bicommissural non-raphe variant (type 0) and the functionally unicuspid variant (type 2, with dual fusion raphe) are rare (Fig. 22.1).

Although aortic valvulopathy (stenosis and/or regurgitation) is the main complication of BAV, aortopathy associated with BAV, such as dilatation of the proximal thoracic aorta, represents a frequent condition, found in approximately 50% of individuals [3, 4].

BAV-related aortopathy can be classified into three different dilatation patterns:

- Type 1: root and ascending aorta dilatation along aortic convexity, typically found in older patients (>50 years); it is associated with coronary cusps fusion (R-L) and aortic valve stenosis.

P. Ciancarella (✉) · V. Bordonaro · A. Secinaro
Department of Imaging, Advanced Cardiovascular Imaging Unit, Bambino Gesù Children's Hospital, IRCCS, Rome, Italy
e-mail: paolo.ciancarella@opbg.net; veronica.bordonaro@opbg.net; aurelio.secinaro@opbg.net

© The Author(s), under exclusive license to Springer Nature Switzerland AG 2024
I. Carbone et al. (eds.), *Imaging of the Aorta*, https://doi.org/10.1007/978-3-031-52527-8_22

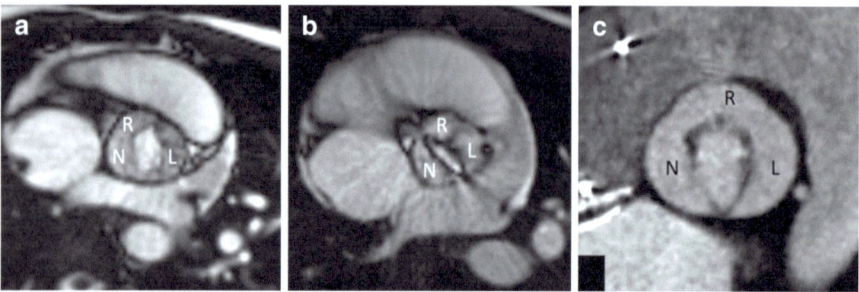

Fig. 22.1 Examples of bicuspid aortic valve: right and non-coronary cusps fusion, type 1 R-N (**a**: 2D cine-SSFP MR image); coronary cusps fusion, type 1 R-L, with thickening and hypomobility of the aortic cusps (**b**: 2D cine-SSFP MR image); functionally monocusp type with two fusion raphe (type2 R-L/R-N) and opening of a single commissure between the left and non-coronary cusps (**c**: CT image)

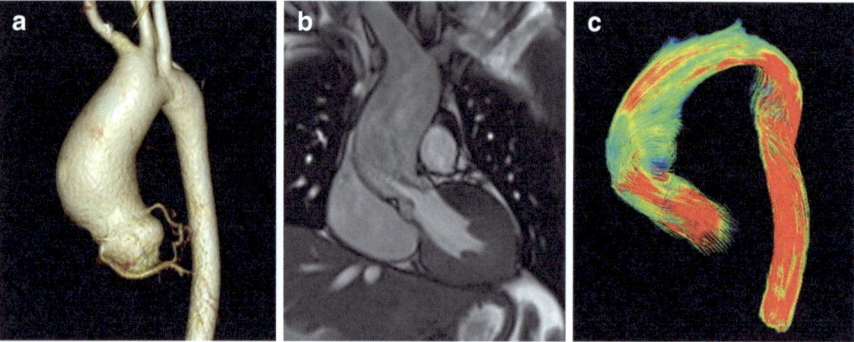

Fig. 22.2 BAV-related aortopathy: dilatation of the tubular tract of the ascending aorta along its convexity (**a**: 3D VR CT reconstruction), with significant aortic stenosis, causing eccentric flow jets directed towards the aortic lateral wall (**b**: 2D cine-SSFP MR image); the helical flow pattern increases parietal stress along the convexity of the ascending aorta (**c**: three-dimensional representation of flow vectors, 4D flow MR image)

- Type 2: isolated dilatation of the ascending aortic tubular tract, with possible involvement of the proximal arch and relative sparing of the aortic root, is typically associated with R-N fusion pattern;
- Type 3: isolated aortic root dilatation, more frequent in younger patients (<40 years), associated with aortic valve regurgitation (Marfan phenotype).

The etiopathogenesis of aortopathy in BAV is multifactorial and results from the interaction between a genetic substrate and hemodynamic mechanisms, such as altered aortic blood flow pattern with abnormal shear force distribution on the arterial wall (wall shear stress). Follow-up of BAV-associated aortopathy involves annual echocardiographic surveillance: if the size of aortic root or ascending aorta is >40 mm or the aortic growth rate is >3 mm/year, further diagnostic investigation by CT/MR is required, with subsequent annual imaging follow-up [5] (Fig. 22.2).

Current guidelines recommend surgical treatment of dilated aortic diseases in patients with BAV in case of aortic size >55 mm; aortic repair is indicated in case of smaller size for BAV patients with risk factors or concomitant valve surgery [5].

Turner Syndrome

Turner syndrome (TS) is a chromosomal disorder caused by partial deletion or monosomy of the X chromosome and occurs in approximately 1 in 2500 live female births. The frequent incidence of cardiovascular disease, such as congenital heart disease, dilatation of the ascending aorta and ischemic heart disease, has a significant impact on life expectancy of individuals with TS [6].

The most common abnormalities of the thoracic aorta involve the aortic arch (about 50% of individuals), with a typical elongated, tortuous and angled morphology of the transverse tract, which is located in a higher position at the thoracic inlet ("gothic arch"). In some cases, aortic kinking is localized to the isthmus, leading to a condition of pseudo-coarctation, without effective narrowing of the vascular lumen [7].

Thoracic aorta dilatation is common in TS, with a prevalence of approximately 40%, and it frequently involves the ascending tract [8].

Aortic dissection represents the main cause of death in young adults with TS, occurring in around 2% of 35 years old women; it affects the ascending tract and the aortic arch in the majority of cases (type A according to Stanford, 63%) while it involves the only descending tract in the remaining cases (type B, 37%).

In Turner syndrome, aortic diameters should be expressed as absolute values and as Aortic Size Index (values indexed to the body surface area, BSA), in order to prevent underestimation of the magnitude of dilatative aortopathy in a population typically characterized by short stature and low BSA values (Fig. 22.3).

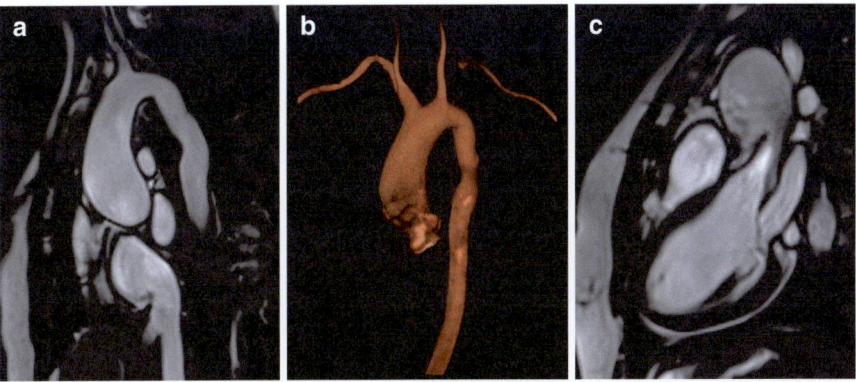

Fig. 22.3 Aortic dilatation in Turner syndrome: the aortic arch has gothic shape without significant stenosis (**a**: 2D cine-SSFP MRI image); the ascending aorta is significantly dilated (considering the aortic size index—ASI, corrected for BSA). Post-surgical disconnection of the left subclavian artery is post-surgical disconnected from the arch, (**b**: 3D VR MR reconstruction); the aortic valve is bicuspid and moderately stenotic (**c**: 2D cine-SSFP MR image)

An ASI >2 cm/m² is considered significant and requires annual surveillance, whereas a caliber >2.5 cm/m² is considered the cut-off value for surgical treatment [9].

Marfan Syndrome

Marfan syndrome (MFS) is a congenital connective tissue disease characterized by multi-organ involvement, including cardiovascular, musculoskeletal, ocular, pulmonary, and skin. It has an autosomal dominant hereditary mechanism and an incidence of approximately 2–3 cases per 10,000 individuals [10].

MFS is caused by mutations in the gene coding for fibrillin-1, an extracellular matrix glycoprotein that is the main constituent of the elastic fibers of various organs and tissues.

Cardiovascular disease represents the main cause of morbidity and mortality in patients with MFS. Dilatation of the ascending aorta is the most frequent manifestation (60–80% of cases), and the development of complications such as dissection and rupture is the leading cause of death in these patients [11].

Dilatation typically involves the aortic root from the annular plane to the sinotubular junction and the proximal ascending tract (annulo-aortic ectasia or pear-shaped aorta) [12]. It is frequently associated with valve regurgitation secondary to the loss of central coaptation of the valve cusps, in the absence of structural abnormalities of the aortic valve (Fig. 22.4).

Surgical treatment in patients with MFS is indicated in case of aortic size >50 mm or for size <50 mm in presence of a family history of dissection, progressive dilatation >2 mm/year, severe mitral or aortic regurgitation, or desire of pregnancy [13].

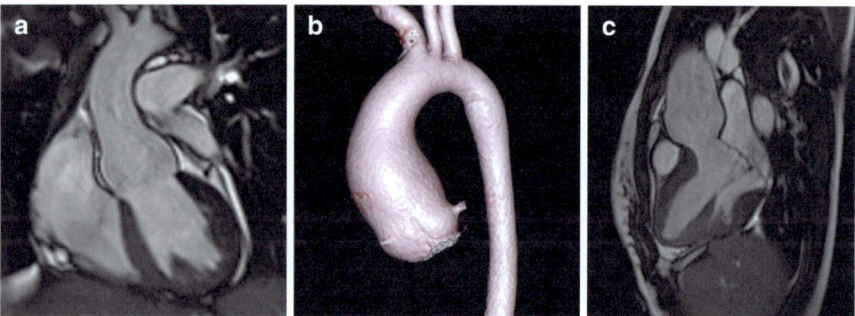

Fig. 22.4 Cardiovascular manifestations in Marfan syndrome: aortic root dilatation with annulus involvement and preserved sino-tubular junction morphology (**a**: 2D cine-SSFP MR image); aortic root and ascending aorta aneurysm with loss of sino-tubular junction (**b**: 3D VR CT reconstruction); mitral annulus dilatation and mitral valve leaflet prolapse with associated regurgitation jet (**c**: 2D cine-SSFP image)

Loeys-Dietz Syndrome

Loeys-Dietz syndrome (LDS) is a rare congenital connective tissue disorder caused by mutations in genes coding for TGF-β receptor types 1 and 2, with an autosomal dominant inheritance mechanism. It is a multisystem disorder that, although it may share some clinical manifestations with MFS and Ehlers-Danlos syndrome type IV, has distinctive phenotypic features and a more aggressive disease course with a significantly lower life expectancy [14]. Cardiovascular manifestations may affect not only the aorta but also the peripheral vascular system. Aortic dilatation can involve the entire thoraco-abdominal axis (a distinguishing feature compared to MFS), also showing a more rapid progression and a higher incidence of complications [15].

For this reason, early treatment of thoracic aortic aneurysms is recommended in LDS, considering a diameter of 4 cm as a surgical cut-off [16].

The involvement of the peripheral vascular system, typically affecting neck arteries but also visceral vessels and coronaries, is characterized by marked tortuosity of the affected vessels, with development of aneurysms or onset of complications even in the absence of vascular dilatation [14].

References

1. Roberts WC. The congenitally bicuspid aortic valve. A study of 85 autopsy cases. Am J Cardiol. 1970;26(1):72–83.
2. Sievers HH, Schmidtke C. A classification system for the bicuspid aortic valve from 304 surgical specimens. J Thorac Cardiovasc Surg. 2007;133:1226–33.
3. Fedak PW, Verma S, David TE, et al. Clinical and pathophysiological implications of a bicuspid aortic valve. Circulation. 2002;106:900–4.
4. Siu SC, Silversides CK. Bicuspid aortic valve disease. J Am Coll Cardiol. 2010;55:2789–800.
5. Erbel R, Aboyans V, Boileau C, et al. ESC Committee for Practice Guidelines. 2014 ESC guidelines on the diagnosis and treatment of aortic diseases: document covering acute and chronic aortic diseases of the thoracic and abdominal aorta of the adult. The Task Force for the Diagnosis and Treatment of Aortic Diseases of the European Society of Cardiology (ESC). Eur Heart J. 2014;35(41):2873–926.
6. Schoemaker MJ, Swerdlow AJ, Higgins CD, et al. Mortality in women with Turner syndrome in Great Britain: a national cohort study. J Clin Endocrinol Metab. 2008;93:4735–42.
7. Sigakis CJG, Browne LP, Bang T, et al. Computed tomography and magnetic resonance imaging of cardiovascular anomalies associated with Turner syndrome. J Thorac Imaging. 2019;34(3):W23–35.
8. Mortensen KH, Hjerrild BE, Stochholm K, et al. Dilation of the ascending aorta in Turner syndrome—a prospective cardiovascular magnetic resonance study. J Cardiovasc Magn Reson. 2011;13(1):24.
9. Matura LA, Ho VB, Rosing DR, et al. Aortic dilatation and dissection in Turner syndrome. Circulation. 2007;116:1663–70.
10. Ammash NM, Sundt TM, Connolly HM. Marfan syndrome—diagnosis and management. Curr Probl Card. 2008;33:7–39.
11. Adams JN, Trent RJ. Aortic complications of Marfan's syndrome. Lancet. 1998;352(9142):1722–3.

12. Stuart AG, Williams A. Marfan's syndrome and the heart. Arch Dis Child. 2007;92(4):351–6.
13. Baumgartner H, Bonhoeffer P, De Groot NM, et al. Task Force on the Management of Grown-up Congenital Heart Disease of the European Society of Cardiology (ESC); Association for European Paediatric Cardiology (AEPC); ESC Committee for Practice Guidelines (CPG). ESC guidelines for the management of grown-up congenital heart disease (new version 2010). Eur Heart J. 2010;31(23):2915–57.
14. Loughborough WW, Minhas KS, Rodrigues JCL, et al. Cardiovascular manifestations and complications of Loeys-Dietz syndrome: CT and MR imaging findings. Radiographics. 2018;38(1):275–86.
15. MacCarrick G, Black JH III, Bowdin S, et al. Loeys-Dietz syndrome: a primer for diagnosis and management. Genet Med. 2014;16(8):576–87.
16. Hiratzka LF, Bakris GL, Beckman JA, et al. 2010 ACCF/AHA/ AATS/ACR/ASA/SCA/SCAI/SIR/STS/SVM guidelines for the diagnosis and management of patients with thoracic aortic disease [...]. J Am Coll Cardiol. 2010;55(14):e27–129.

Congenital Obstructive Heart Disease

23

Paolo Ciancarella, Veronica Bordonaro, and Aurelio Secinaro

Aortic Coarctation

Aortic coarctation (CoA) accounts for 5–8% of all congenital heart disease, with an incidence of 4 per 1000 live births and a predominance in males [1].

It can occur as an isolated anomaly or be associated with other congenital cardiovascular malformations, including bicuspid aortic valve and aortic arch hypoplasia.

CoA is a focal narrowing of the aortic lumen at the isthmic site that is the aortic tract between the origin of the left subclavian artery and the insertion of the ductus arteriosus. Narrowing typically occurs in the juxtaductal site, with a deep parietal incision at the level of the aortic isthmus opposite the insertion of the ductus arteriosus (posterior shelf).

CoA corrective treatment is indicated in patients with arterial hypertension and a pressure gradient >20 mmHg between upper and lower limbs or a caliber reduction at the site of stenosis ≥50% compared to the reference diameter of the aorta measured at the diaphragm [2].

Treatment options vary according to the age of the patient: surgical treatment is indicated in infants, whereas an endovascular approach is preferred in adults.

The need for re-intervention for recurrence of coarctation is frequent in these patients (4–14% of subjects) and it is caused by residual ductal tissue, post-surgical fibrosis, residual aortic arch hypoplasia, and intrastent re-stenosis from neointimal hyperplasia [3].

Transthoracic echocardiography represents the first diagnostic modality in the suspicion of CoA and it is usually sufficient in the neonatal period to correctly

---

P. Ciancarella · V. Bordonaro (✉) · A. Secinaro
Department of Imaging, Advanced Cardiovascular Imaging Unit, Bambino Gesù Children's Hospital, IRCCS, Rome, Italy
e-mail: paolo.ciancarella@opbg.net; veronica.bordonaro@opbg.net; aurelio.secinaro@opbg.net

establish the diagnosis and plan treatment. CT is the second-line method in cases in which is required an accurate definition of the aortic arch anatomy and the extension of the collateral circles of the chest wall (Fig. 23.1). CT is also useful in postoperative follow-up (Fig. 23.2), in particular to evaluate patients undergoing interventional procedures with stent placement [4].

MRI has limited use in the diagnostic phase, as it may be useful in rare cases with late diagnosis of CoA, while it is the preferred diagnostic technique in postoperative follow-up. In fact, MRI can provide not only anatomical but also functional/hemodynamic information.

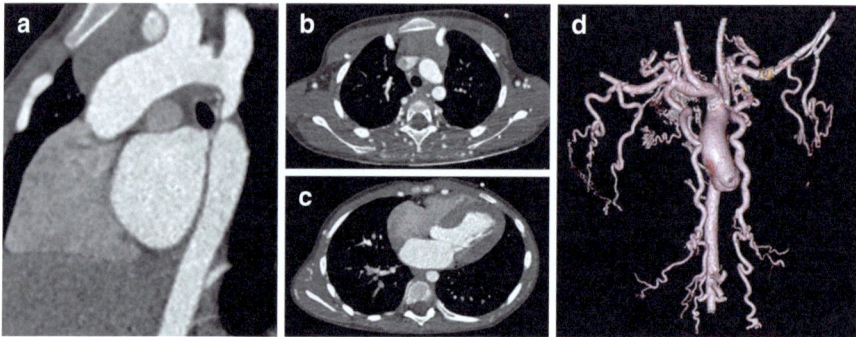

Fig. 23.1 Severe aortic coarctation with posterior iuxta-ductal shelf and severe aortic isthmus stenosis (**a**: sagittal MPR CT reconstruction). Extensive collateral vessels of the thoracic wall, with marked hypertrophy of internal mammary arteries, intercostal branches and paravertebral vessels; significant concentric left ventricle hypertrophy, due to pressure overload (**b**, **c**: axial CT images); the 3D VR image clearly shows the extension of collateral wall circles, indicative of severe isthmic coarctation (**d**)

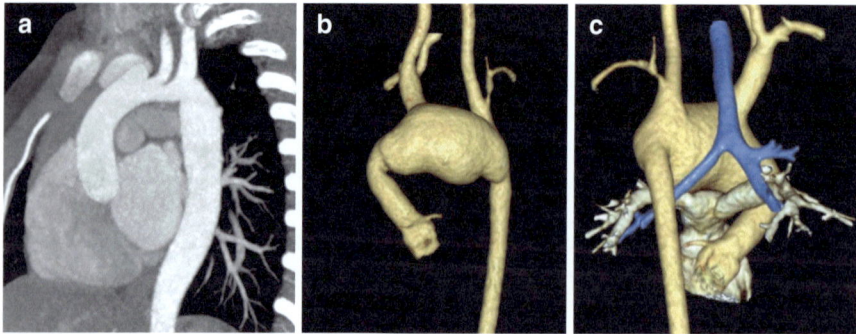

Fig. 23.2 Post-coartectomy CT follow-up: moderate hypoplasia of the transverse aortic arch after end-to-end anastomosis, with post-isthmic descending aorta dilatation (**a**: sagittal MIP reconstruction). Marked dilatation of the aortic arch after patch enlargement, with post-surgical left subclavian artery stenosis (**b**: 3D VR reconstruction). The pulmonary trunk, main pulmonary arteries and left main bronchus are compressed by the aortic arch aneurysm (**c**: 3D VR CT reconstruction)

Williams Syndrome

Williams syndrome (WS) is a genetic disorder that affects approximately 1 in 10,000 live births and involves multiple systems, including cardiovascular, central nervous, and connective tissue systems [5].

This syndrome is caused by a deletion on the long arm of chromosome 7, resulting in a defect in elastin synthesis. This leads to a loss of elasticity and thickening of the tunica media of the vascular wall as well as hypertrophy of smooth muscle cells. These histopathological alterations cause the typical cardiovascular manifestations of WS, such as supravalvular aortic stenosis, aortic arch, and/or thoracoabdominal aorta hypoplasia and pulmonary arteries stenosis [6].

Supravalvular aortic stenosis is the most common cardiovascular anomaly and it is found in 70% of individuals with WS. The narrowing is typically located at the level of the sinotubular junction and leads to a characteristic "hourglass" morphology of the proximal thoracic aorta (Fig. 23.3).

The coronary ostia are often situated close to the supravalvular obstruction, with consequent exposure to high pressures during the systolic phase and possible development of parietal fibrosis, tunica media hypertrophy, and coronary stenosis. Additionally, the aortic valve cusps are frequently thickened and may be partially fused with the supravalvular ridge, potentially leading to coronary hooding and altered myocardial perfusion. In some cases, supravalvular stenosis may be accompanied by varying degrees of thoracic aorta hypoplasia, most commonly in the

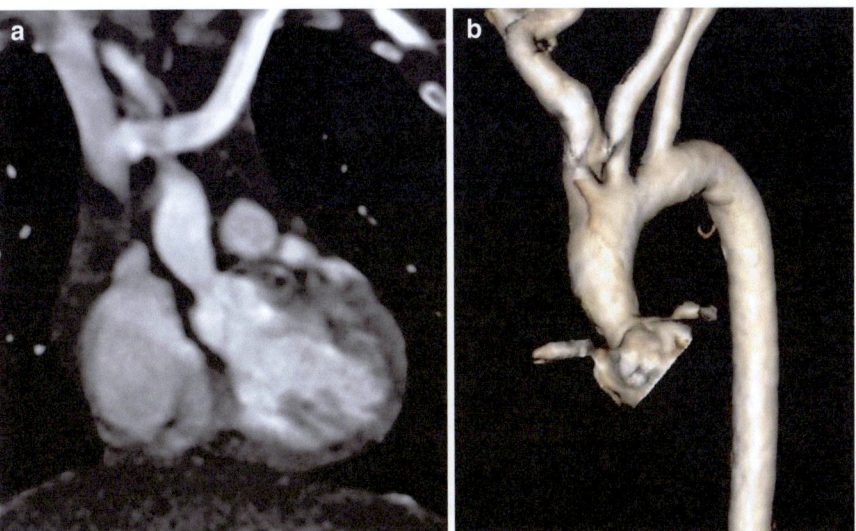

Fig. 23.3 Supravalvular aortic stenosis in Williams syndrome: focal narrowing of the proximal ascending aorta (**a**: coronal MPR CT reconstruction), with normal caliber of the other aortic tracts (**b**: 3D VR CT reconstruction)

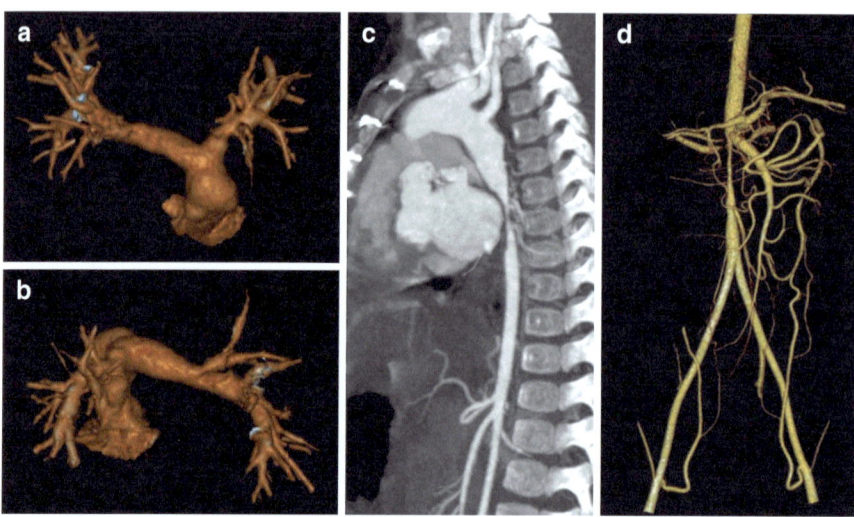

Fig. 23.4 Other cardiovascular manifestations in Williams syndrome: hypoplasia of the main pulmonary arteries and multiple intraparenchinal branches stenosis (**a, b**: 3D VR CT reconstruction); marked segmental narrowing of the middle descending thoracic aorta (**c**: sagittal MIP CT reconstruction); severe hypoplasia of the abdominal aorta (mid-aortic syndrome), involving the proximal visceral arterial branches (**d**: 3D VR CT reconstruction) with collateral circulation of the abdominal wall (inferior epigastric arteries) and splanchnic arterial vessels connections (Riolan's arch)

aortic arch. Hypoplasia of the distal thoracic and abdominal aorta, also known as mid-aortic syndrome, is often associated with visceral arteries stenosis (celiac trunk, mesenteric arteries, and renal arteries) and collateral compensatory circles hypertrophy (arch of Riolano, etc.) (Fig. 23.4).

Pulmonary arteries stenosis is another common cardiovascular manifestation in WS, affecting around 45% of individuals. Stenoses may be single or multiple and can involve the pulmonary branches diffusely [7].

References

1. Singh S, Hakim FA, Sharma A, et al. Hypoplasia, pseudocoarctation and coarctation of the aorta—a systematic review. Heart Lung Circ. 2015;24:110–8.
2. Baumgartner H, Bonhoeffer P, De Groot NM, et al. Task Force on the Management of Grown-up Congenital Heart Disease of the European Society of Cardiology (ESC); Association for EuropeanPaediatric Cardiology (AEPC); ESC Committee for Practice Guidelines (CPG). ESC guidelines for the management of grown-up congenital heart disease (new version 2010). Eur Heart J. 2010;31(23):2915–57.
3. Dijkema EJ, Leiner T, Grotenhuis HB. Diagnosis, imaging and clinical management of aortic coarctation. Heart. 2017;103(15):1148–55.
4. Ciancarella P, Ciliberti P, Santangelo TP, et al. Noninvasive imaging of congenital cardiovascular defects. Radiol Med. 2020;25(11):1167–85.

5. Pober BR. Williams-Beuren syndrome. N Engl J Med. 2010;362:239–52.
6. Wessel A, Gravenhorst V, Buchhorn R, et al. Risk of sudden death in the Williams-Beuren syndrome. Am J Med Genet A. 2004;127A(3):234–7.
7. Das KM, Momenah TS, Larsson SG, et al. Williams-Beuren syndrome: computed tomography imaging review. Pediatr Cardiol. 2014;35(8):1309–20.

Anatomical Variants and Congenital Anomalies of the Aortic Arch

24

Paolo Ciancarella, Veronica Bordonaro, and Aurelio Secinaro

Aortic arch anomalies represent a broad spectrum of malformations involving the position/laterality of the arch, the pattern of origin, ramification, and course of the vessels originating from it.

There are three types of aortic arch based on its position and course: left arch, right arch, and double arch. The definition of a right or left arch refers to the side of the trachea with respect to which it is located when it crosses a main bronchus (right or left) and not to the hemilateral of the thorax in which the ascending aorta is positioned. The trachea usually appears slightly deviated toward the side opposite the arch [1].

The aortic arch normally and most frequently courses left-posterior and gives rise to three branches: the first is the brachiocephalic trunk (or innominate trunk), which gives rise to the right common carotid artery and the right subclavian artery, the second is the left common carotid artery and the third is the left subclavian artery [2].

Aortic arch anomalies have a prevalence that varies between 1% and 2% of the general population [3]. They include forms that clinically manifest themselves already in the neonatal period, as they can determine tracheal compression (so-called vascular rings), as well as being associated with heart diseases and/or chromosomal abnormalities [4].

A vascular ring is formed when a vessel (or an atretic portion of it) completely or incompletely surrounds the trachea and the esophagus, leading to the development of respiratory distress in the case of tracheal compression, and dysphagia and/or regurgitation in the case of esophageal compression. Direct airways compression can lead to tracheobronchomalacia, defined as a weakening of the tracheal rings with collapse of the lumen during the expiratory phase, which can sometimes persist despite surgical correction of the vascular ring [5].

P. Ciancarella · V. Bordonaro · A. Secinaro (✉)
Advanced Cardiothoracic Imaging Unit, Bambino Gesù Children's Hospital, IRCCS, Rome, Italy
e-mail: paolo.ciancarella@opbg.net; veronica.bordonaro@opbg.net; aurelio.secinaro@opbg.net

© The Author(s), under exclusive license to Springer Nature Switzerland AG 2024
I. Carbone et al. (eds.), *Imaging of the Aorta*,
https://doi.org/10.1007/978-3-031-52527-8_24

However, this broad spectrum of abnormalities also includes clinically silent forms that may represent an incidental finding in adulthood.

Embryology

The etiology of aortic arch development abnormalities is closely related to the complex stages of embryogenesis and their proper sequence during the fetal period [3, 4].

During the third week of gestation, the primitive aorta consists of a dorsal and ventral segment, between which six pairs of primitive arches develop (numbered cranio-caudally). The normal appearance of the mature aortic arch develops by the regression of some arches and the persistence of others, according to a mechanism of cell migration that is not yet fully understood. In particular, the third, fourth, and sixth arches are the main arches that contribute to the formation of the mature aortic arch and its branches. The third arch forms the common carotid artery and a segment of the internal carotid arteries, while the fourth forms the definitive aortic arch. The ventral portion of the sixth arch forms the distal segments of the pulmonary artery, while from its dorsal portion develops the ductus arteriosus [6].

The abnormal persistence and/or involution of these arches explain the etiology of most of the aortic arch morphology included in this wide spectrum of anomalies.

Imaging

In case of suspected aortic arch anomalies, echocardiography is the preferred non-invasive imaging method, particularly in pediatric patients. However, especially in patients with complex anatomy, CT and MRI represent the methods of choice for a detailed analysis of the vascular anatomy and for a pre-surgical evaluation of the relationships of vessels to the airway and esophagus [1, 7].

More specifically, CT angiography represents the preferred technique for its high spatial resolution, allowing a detailed evaluation of vascular anatomy and other intrathoracic structures, through the use of multiplanar images with 3D volume rendering reconstructions and three-dimensional intracavitary visualization (virtual bronchoscopy) [8, 9].

In pediatric patients, CT also allows the acquisition of spontaneous breathing sequential images for a dynamic assessment of airway compression.

Left Aortic Arch

Anatomical Variants

Common Origin of Brachiocephalic Trunk and Left Common Carotid Artery ("Bovine" Aortic Arch)

This anomaly is characterized by the common origin of the brachiocephalic trunk and left common carotid artery and is the most common variant of aortic branchies, which is found in approximately 13% of the population. However, the term "bovine arch" is misleading because in animals there is a single common branch from which all aortic vessels originate [10].

Although initially considered clinically insignificant, this variant has recently been linked to an increased risk of thoracic aortic aneurysms due to the presence of only two fixation points instead of the usual three [3].

Variants of Vertebral Artery Origin

The direct origin of the left vertebral artery from the arch is a common finding in autopsies (5% of cases) and is clinically insignificant. However, its presence is noteworthy as it may have implications in cases of aortic surgery.

Congenital Anomalies

Left Aortic Arch with Aberrant Right Subclavian Artery (Lusoria)

This is the most common congenital anomaly, with a prevalence of approximately 0.5–2% [4, 7]. In this anomaly, the right common carotid artery originates as the first vessel in the aortic arch, followed by the left common carotid artery and the left subclavian artery. The right subclavian artery originates as the last branch from the proximal descending aorta and crosses the mediastinum from left to right, passing posteriorly to the esophagus and trachea (Fig. 24.1).

This anomaly is generally asymptomatic as it is not associated with a vascular ring. However, in 10% of cases, it may cause esophageal compression, defined as "dysphagia lusoria," which can be confirmed by an esophagogram with barium.

Left Aortic Arch with Right Subclavian Artery Originating from Retroesophageal Diverticulum

This is an anomaly characterized by the origin of the aberrant right subclavian artery from a blind diverticular structure with a retroesophageal course, known as Kommerell diverticulum. It represents a remnant of the dorsal arch, which develops

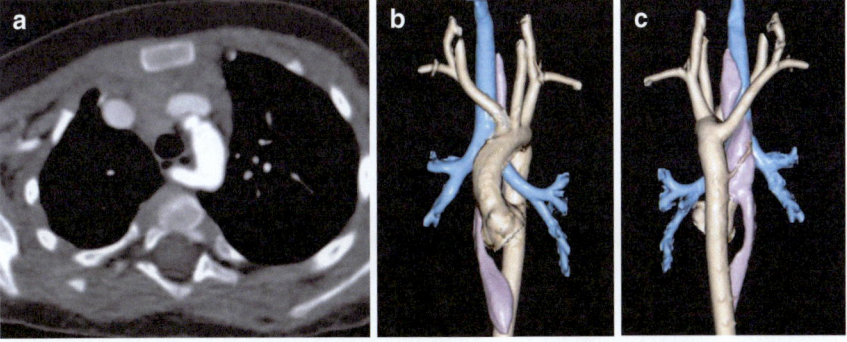

Fig. 24.1 Contrast-enhanced CT image in oblique axial projection (**a**) with MIP reconstruction and 3D VR reconstructions of the aortic arch, airway and esophagus (**b**, **c**) in patient with left aortic arch and right subclavian retroesophageal artery, without Kommerell diverticulum

as a consequence of persistence of the right VI arch. This results in the development of a vascular ring, complemented by the right ductus arteriosus or ligamentum arteriosus. As a general rule, in the presence of a retroesophageal diverticulum, the ductus arteriosus/ligamentum arteriosus is located opposite the aortic arch and originates from the junction between the diverticulum and the subclavian artery [3, 4].

Right Aortic Arch

Right aortic arch represents a rare anomaly, with an incidence of approximately 0.1% of the population [11]. This anomaly has been classified into three subtypes, based on the aortic arch branching pattern: type I, right aortic arch with mirror image branching pattern; type II, right arch with retroesophageal left subclavian artery; and type III, a very rare form of right arch with isolated subclavian artery [7].

Type I: Right Aortic Arch with Mirror Image Branching Pattern

In this anomaly, the aortic arch branches originate exactly specular to that of the normal left arch; therefore, the first branch to originate is the left brachiocephalic trunk, followed by the right common carotid artery and the right subclavian artery (Fig. 24.2, Panel 1). It results from involution of the dorsal segment of the left aortic arch between the left subclavian artery and descending aorta (left IV branchial arch), as well as the ductus arteriosus, in a hypothetical double aortic arch.

This anomaly does not typically form a vascular ring; however, it is frequently associated with congenital heart diseases, such as tetralogy of Fallot, truncus arteriosus, tricuspid atresia, or transposition of the great vessels with pulmonary stenosis. It is often present in cases of chromosomal abnormalities such as 22q11 deletion syndrome.

Rarely, it may be associated with the presence of a left-sided ductus arteriosus between the pulmonary artery and a left retroesophageal diverticulum, resulting in a vascular ring, with possible development of tracheo-bronchial compression phenomena (Fig. 24.2, Panel 2).

Type II: Right Aortic Arch with Retroesophageal Left Subclavian Artery

This is the most common subtype of right arch and contrary to type I, it is only rarely associated with congenital heart diseases [12].

In this anomaly, the first vessel originating from the right arch is the right common carotid artery, followed by the right subclavian artery, whereas the left subclavian artery originates as the last branch and shows an oblique retroesophageal course, from the right caudal to the left cranial side.

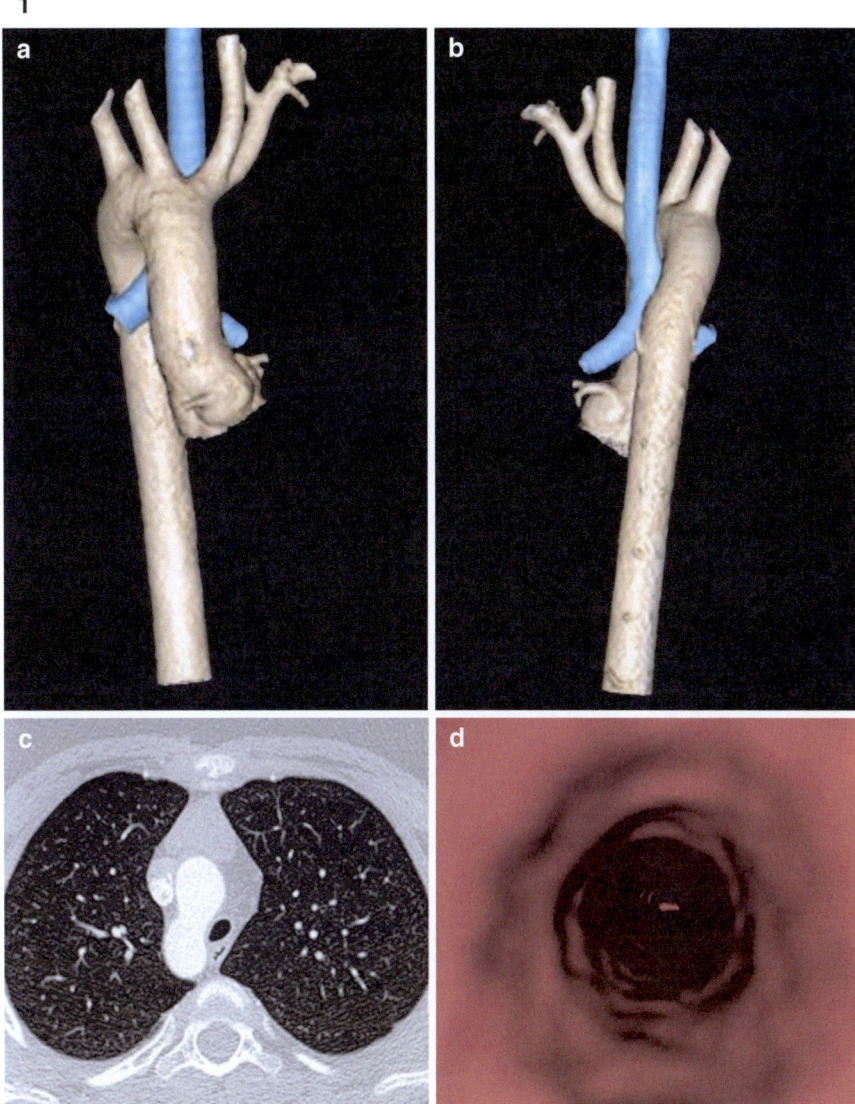

Fig. 24.2 *Panel 1*: right aortic arch with mirror image branching pattern. (**a, b**) 3D VR reconstructions of the aorta and airways; (**c**) axial CT image with lung window and virtual bronchoscopy reconstruction; (**d**) demonstrating only slight tracheal compression due to the aortic arch. *Panel 2*: right aortic arch with mirror image branching pattern and retroesophageal diverticulum. (**a, b**) 3D VR reconstructions of the aorta and airways; (**c**) axial CT image with lung window and virtual bronchoscopy reconstruction (**d**) demonstrating marked extrinsic tracheal lumen narrowing

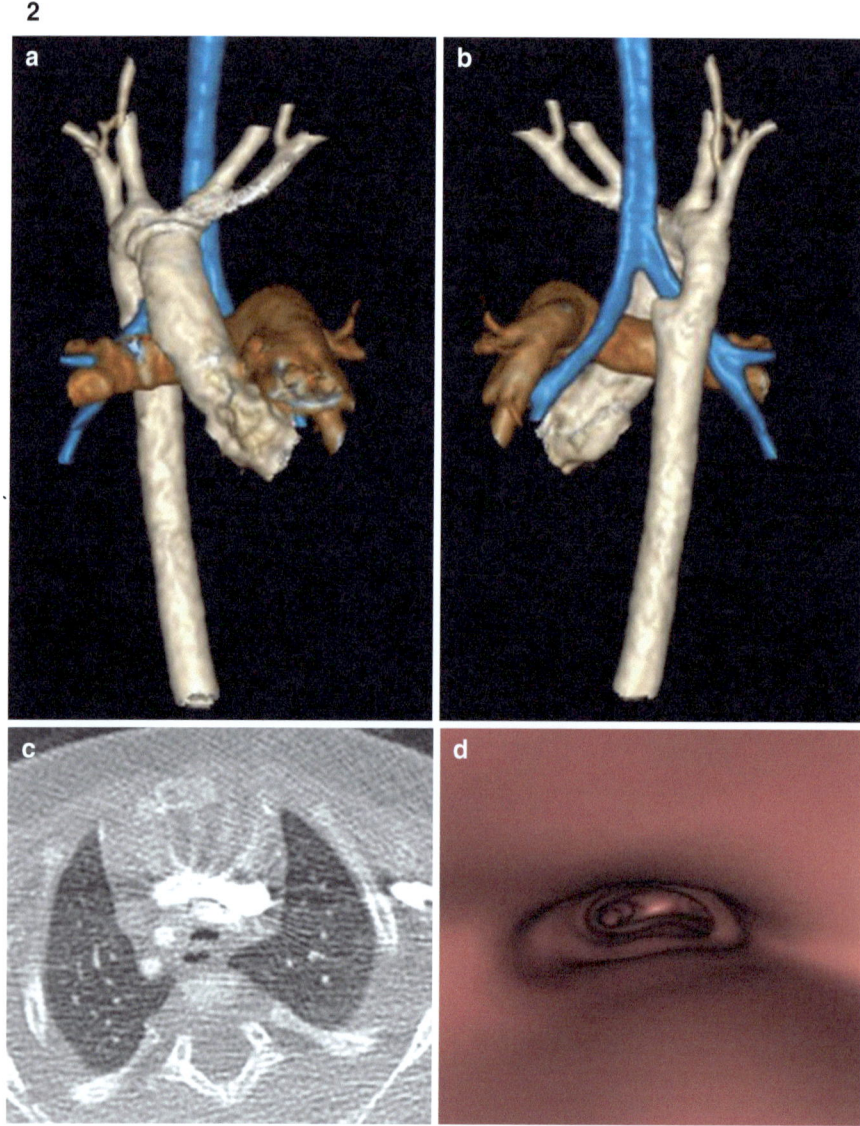

Fig. 24.2 (continued)

It results from the involution of the left IV arch between the left subclavian artery and the left common carotid artery and is not associated with the formation of a vascular ring, since the ductus arteriosus is located on the right side.

In cases where the described anomaly is associated with the persistence of the left VI arch, the left subclavian artery will emerge from the remnant of the left

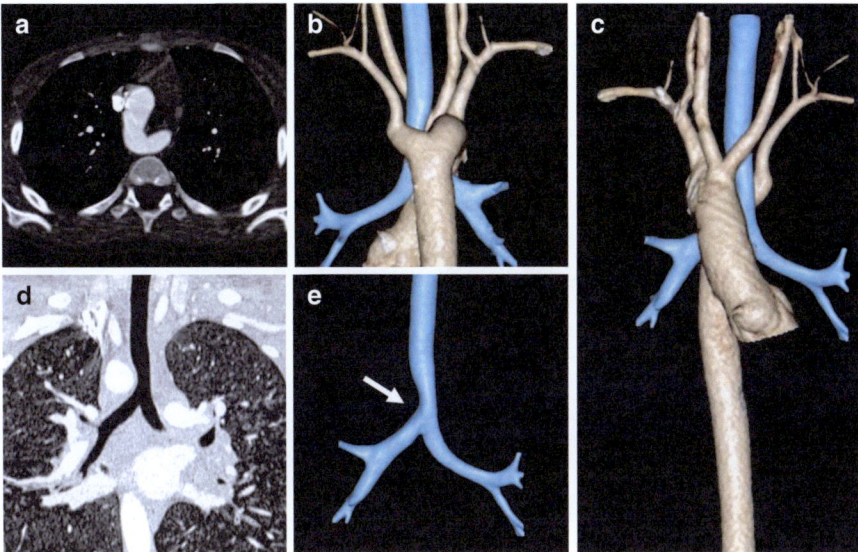

Fig. 24.3 Right aortic arch with retroesophageal left subclavian artery and Kommerell diverticulum. Contrast enhanced axial CT image (**a**) and 3D VR reconstruction of aorta and airways in posterior (**b**) and anterior (**c**) views show the retroesophageal diverticulum and the aberrant left subclavian artery. Coronal CT image (**d**) and VR reconstruction (**e**) show the tracheal wall compression due to the vascular ring (arrow)

dorsal arch, which forms the retroesophageal diverticulum of Kommerell. This arrangement results in a vascular ring around the trachea and esophagus, completed laterally by the left duct/arterial ligament (Fig. 24.3).

Double Arch

Double arch is an anomaly characterized by the persistence of the right and left IV branchial arches, forming a complete vascular ring around the trachea and esophagus; each arch separately gives rise to the common carotid artery and the subclavian artery of the ipsilateral side (Fig. 24.4).

Clinically, tracheo-oesophageal compression is characterized by symptoms such as stridor, recurrent respiratory infections, dysphagia and regurgitation, which appear within the first 6 months of life [13].

In approximately 75% of cases, the right arch is dominant, the descending thoracic aorta is left-posterior, and the ductus arteriosus is located on the left.

In contrast, the left aortic arch is usually hypoplastic or completely atretic. In the latter case, differentiation between double arch with atretic left portion and right aortic arch with mirror image branching pattern may be difficult [3].

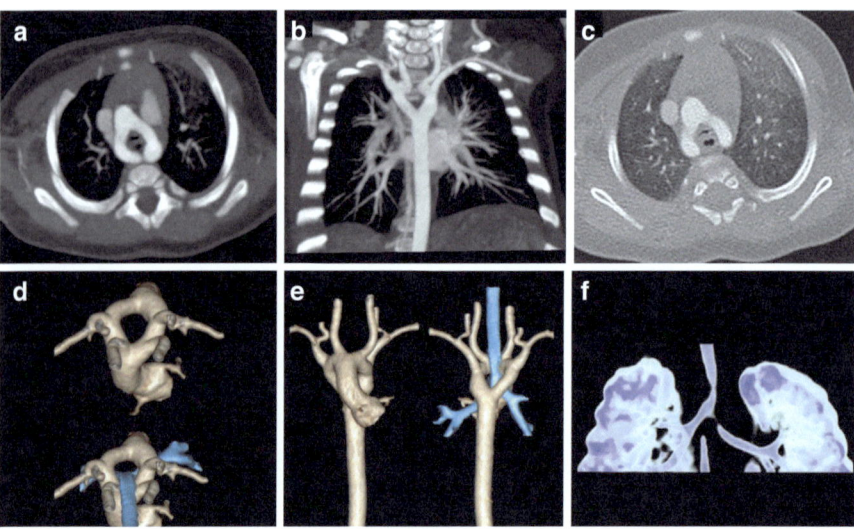

Fig. 24.4 CT images with MIP reconstruction in axial (**a**) and coronal oblique (**b**) and related 3D VR reconstructions with top view (**d**) and anterior/posterior view (**e**) of a patient with balanced double arch forming a complete vascular ring around trachea and esophagus. In the axial CT image with lung parenchyma finger (**c**) and dynamic 3D airway reconstruction (**f**), airway compression at the site of the vascular ring is appreciated, characterized by imprint on the right lateral wall of the trachea and filiform lumen of the proximal left main bronchus

Cervical Arch

In this condition, the aortic arch is located at an abnormally high position in the upper mediastinum, reaching or extending above the level of the clavicles [4].

The most frequent vascular setting is characterized by right aortic arch reaching the thoracic inlet, with separate origin of the common carotid arteries, presence of contralateral subclavian artery aberrant from aortic diverticulum, and retroesophageal descending aorta running contralaterally to the side of the aortic arch (Fig. 24.5).

Most patients do not require surgical correction as the anomaly does not cause compression symptoms. However, it may be associated with intracardiac defects and genetic syndromes such as 22q11 microdeletion.

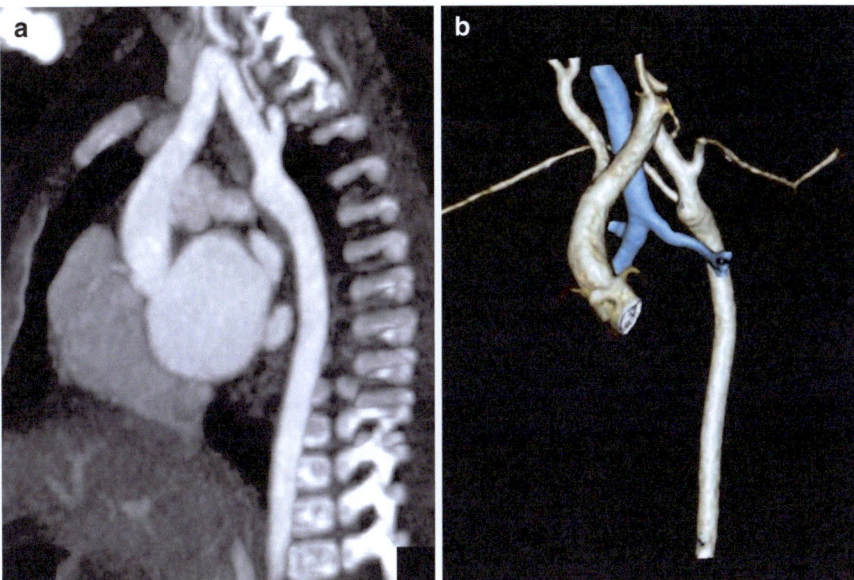

Fig. 24.5 MIP reconstruction (**a**) and volume rendering reconstruction (**b**) of a Left cervical aortic arch extending above the level of the clavicles, with gothic morphology and kinking of the transverse tract. The aortic branching pattern is characterized by right common carotid artery with distal origin from ascending aorta and aberrant right subclavian artery with retroesophageal course, without Kommerell diverticulum

References

1. Weinberg PM. Aortic arch anomalies. J Cardiovasc Magn Reson. 2006;8(4):633–43.
2. Tawfik AM, Sobh DM, Ashamallah GA, et al. Prevalence and types of aortic arch variants and anomalies in congenital heart diseases. Acad Radiol. 2019;26(7):930–6.
3. Priya S, Thomas R, Nagpal P, et al. Congenital anomalies of the aortic arch. Cardiovasc Diagn Ther. 2018;8(Suppl 1):S26–44.
4. Hanneman K, Newman B, Chan F. Congenital variants and anomalies of the aortic arch. Radiographics. 2017;37(1):32–51.
5. Carden KA, Boiselle PM, Waltz DA, Ernst A. Tracheomalacia and tracheobronchomalacia in children and adults: an in-depth review. Chest. 2005;127(3):984–1005.
6. Kau T, Sinzig M, Gasser J, et al. Aortic development and anomalies. Semin Intervent Radiol. 2007;24(2):141–52.
7. Türkvatan A, Büyükbayraktar FG, Olçer T, Cumhur T. Congenital anomalies of the aortic arch: evaluation with the use of multidetector computed tomography. Korean J Radiol. 2009;10(2):176–84.
8. Maldonado JA, Henry T, Gutiérrez FR. Congenital thoracic vascular anomalies. Radiol Clin North Am. 2010;48(1):85–115.
9. Schertler T, Wildermuth S, Teodorovic N, et al. Visualization of congenital thoracic vascular anomalies using multi-detector row computed tomography and two- and three-dimensional post-processing. Eur J Radiol. 2007;61(1):97–119.

10. Layton KF, Kallmes DF, Cloft HJ, et al. Bovine aortic arch variant in humans: clarification of a common misnomer. AJNR Am J Neuroradiol. 2006;27(7):1541–2.
11. D'Antonio F, Khalil A, Zidere V, Carvalho JS. Fetuses with right aortic arch: a multicenter cohort study and meta-analysis. Ultrasound Obstet Gynecol. 2016;47(4):423–32.
12. Cinà CS, Althani H, Pasenau J, Abouzahr L. Kommerell's diverticulum and right-sided aortic arch: a cohort study and review of the literature. J Vasc Surg. 2004;39(1):131–9.
13. Gould SW, Rigsby CK, Donnelly LF, et al. Useful signs for the assessment of vascular rings on cross-sectional imaging. Pediatr Radiol. 2015;45(13):2004–16.

Part VIII

Taking It to the Test

Clinical Cases

25

Federica Giulio, Elena Orlando, Alessandro Onori, Simone Ciaglia, Bianca Rocco, Pier Giorgio Nardis, Davide Curione, Nunzia Di Meo, and Teresa Falcone

---

F. Giulio · E. Orlando
Department of Radiological, Oncological and Pathological Sciences, "Sapienza" University of Rome, I.C.O.T. Hospital, Latina, LT, Italy

A. Onori
Academic Diagnostic Imaging Division, Faculty of Pharmacy and Medicine, Department of Medical-Surgical Sciences and Biotechnologies, University of Rome "Sapienza",
I.C.O.T. Hospital, Latina, Italy
e-mail: alessandro.onori@uniroma1.it

S. Ciaglia · B. Rocco · P. G. Nardis (✉)
Vascular and Interventional Radiology Unit, Department of Radiological, Oncological and Anathomo-Pathological Science, Policlinico Umberto I, "Sapienza" University of Rome, Rome, Italy
e-mail: p.nardis@policlinicoumberto1.it

D. Curione
Advanced Cardiovascular Imaging Unit, Department of Imaging, Bambino Gesù Children's Hospital, IRCCS, Rome, Italy
e-mail: davide.curione@opbg.net

N. Di Meo · T. Falcone
Department of Medical and Surgical Specialties, Radiological Sciences, and Public Health, University of Brescia, Brescia, Italy

Radiology Unit 2, ASST Spedali Civili di Brescia, Brescia, Italy
e-mail: n.dimeo@unibs.it; t.falcone@unibs.it

© The Author(s), under exclusive license to Springer Nature Switzerland AG 2024
I. Carbone et al. (eds.), *Imaging of the Aorta*,
https://doi.org/10.1007/978-3-031-52527-8_25

Case 1

Federica Giulio

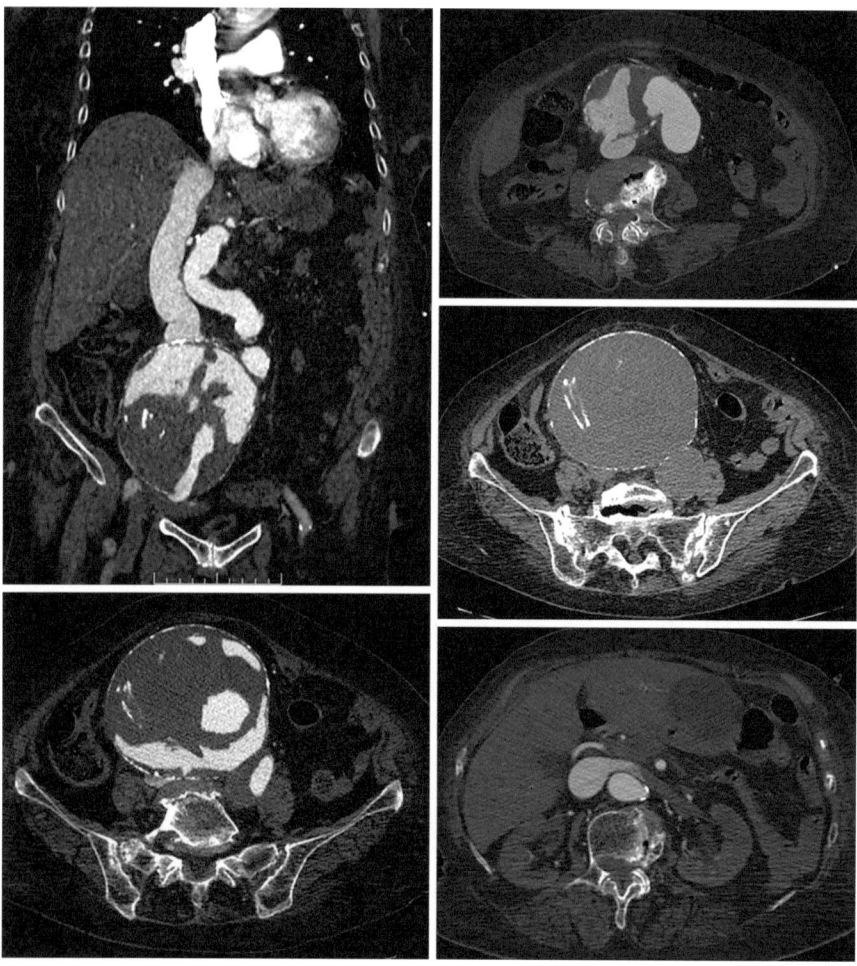

1. Choose the correct initial imaging examination when an abdominal aortic aneurysm complication is suspected:
    (a) Multiphase multidetector CT angiography
    (b) Angiography
    (c) Nonenhanced CT
    (d) Color Doppler ultrasonography
2. Which site of the aortic wall is most commonly involved in abdominal aneurysm complication?
    (a) Postero-lateral
    (b) Antero-lateral

25 Clinical Cases

   (c) Posterior
   (d) Anterior
3. The case shown in the images above is
   (a) Aortoenteric fistula
   (b) Aortic dissection
   (c) Aortocaval fistula
   (d) Micotic abdominal aortic aneurysm
4. Which indirect signs of aortocaval fistula can you find in the images above?
   (a) Draped aorta sign
   (b) Loss of the flat plane between aorta and IVC
   (c) Late kidneys enhancement
   (d) Simultaneous opacification of the aorta and the renal veins
5. Which is the most important CT diagnostic sign of aortocaval fistula?
   (a) Poor perfusion of kidneys
   (b) Simultaneous presence of contrast in aorta and IVC during the arterial phase
   (c) Enlargement of the IVC
   (d) Thrombus fissuration
6. Which other signs of aneurysm rupture can you find in the imaging above?
   (a) Hyperattenuating crescent sign
   (b) Focal wall discontinuity
   (c) Periaortic stranding
   (d) Retroperitoneal hematoma

Answers
1. (a)
2. (a)
3. (c)
4. (b)
5. (b)
6. (b)

Case 2

Elena Orlando

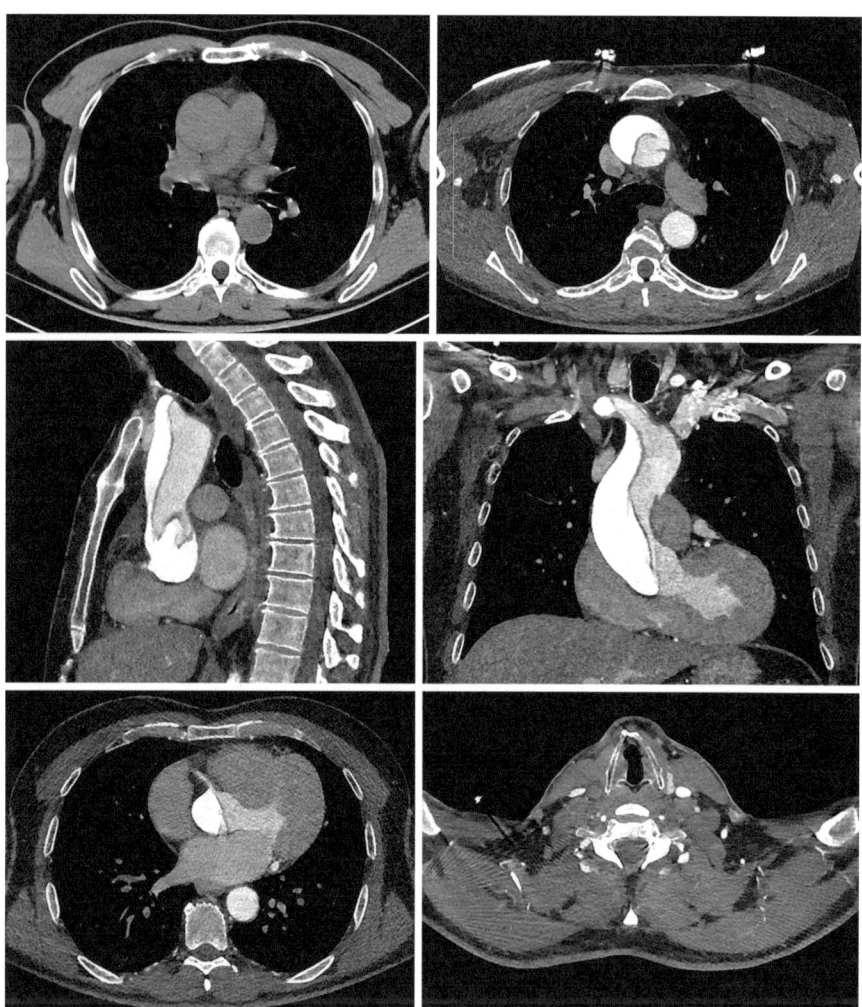

1. The exam shown is:
   (a) A chest CT angiography for the study of pulmonary circulation
   (b) A venous phase chest CT
   (c) A gated-CT angiography
   (d) A non-gated chest CT angiography
2. The case shown in the figure is:
   (a) An aneurysm of the aortic arch
   (b) A Stanford B dissection
   (c) A DeBakey III dissection
   (d) A Stanford A dissection

3. The real lumen:
   (a) Is often thrombosed in chronic dissections
   (b) Has higher contrast density than the false lumen
   (c) Has lower contrast density than the false lumen
   (d) Has the same contrast density as the false lumen
4. The false lumen:
   (a) Generally has larger dimensions than the true lumen
   (b) Generally has smaller dimensions than the true lumen
   (c) Is recognizable by the presence of parietal calcifications
   (d) Is not always visible in acute dissections
5. The right coronary arises:
   (a) From the true lumen
   (b) From the false lumen
   (c) From both true and false lumens
   (d) The origin of the right coronary artery is not involved in the dissection
6. The dissection flap:
   (a) Does not involve epiaortic trunks
   (b) Involves the anonymous trunk and occludes the right carotid
   (c) Occludes the left carotid artery
   (d) Involves the right carotid and vertebral artery
7. The dissection flap:
   (a) Originates at the aortic valve plane
   (b) Is fixed in both systole and diastole
   (c) Does not involve the aortic arch
   (d) Involves the aortic arch and the descending aorta
8. The exit breach:
   (a) Is not viewable
   (b) Is located at the aortic arch
   (c) Is located in along the left carotid
   (d) Is located in along the descending aorta
9. Considering the radiological findings, which symptoms is the Patient is most likely to present:
   (a) Chest pain and left side deficit
   (b) Hemoptysis
   (c) Hemoptoe
   (d) Stable angin

Answers
1. (c)
2. (d)
3. (b)
4. (a)
5. (c)
6. (b)
7. (a)
8. (a)
9. (a)

Case 3

Alessandro Onori

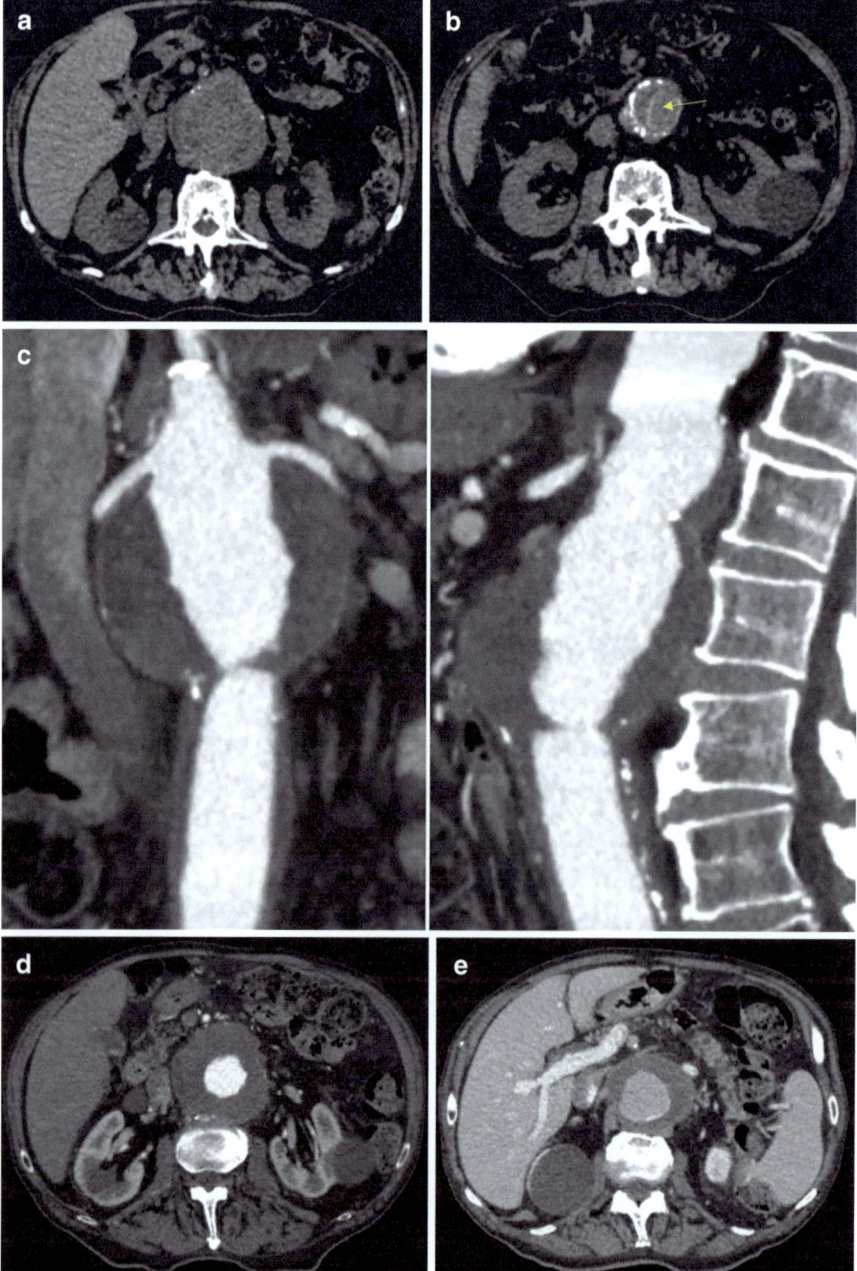

25 Clinical Cases

1. *Unenhanced CT scan*:
   (a) Can be useful in the evaluation of aortic aneurysms
   (b) May help in detecting an impending rupture
   (c) Can be replaced by virtual unenhanced imaging at Dual Energy CT
   (d) All of the above
2. *Figure a shows*:
   (a) Well-defined peripheral and circumferential crescent of increased attenuation
   (b) Periaortic fat stranding
   (c) Vertebral body bone remodeling
   (d) Periaortic air bubbles
3. *The arrow in Fig. b indicates*:
   (a) Displaced parietal calcifications in central lumen
   (b) Focal gap in circumferential wall calcifications
   (c) Calcified intramural hematoma
   (d) Aortic prosthesis
4. *Figure c demonstrates*:
   (a) Subrenal abdominal aortic aneurysm
   (b) Renal arteries originate from the aneurysm sac
   (c) Fusiform aneurysm
   (d) a + c
5. *In Fig. d*:
   (a) Impending rupture can be suspected
   (b) The posterior wall of the aorta is not identifiable as distinct from the contour of adjacent vertebral bodies (*draped aorta sign*)
   (c) Signs of aortic aneurysm inflammation are shown
   (d) a + b
6. *The venous phase shown in Fig. e*:
   (a) Shows blood pooling of the aneurysm sac
   (b) Identifies an aortocaval fistula
   (c) Demonstrates aortic wall rupture on the right posterior side
   (d) None of the above

Answers
1. (d)
2. (a)
3. (d)
4. (d)
5. (d)
6. (d)

Case 4

Simone Ciaglia Bianca Rocco, and Pier Giorgio Nardis

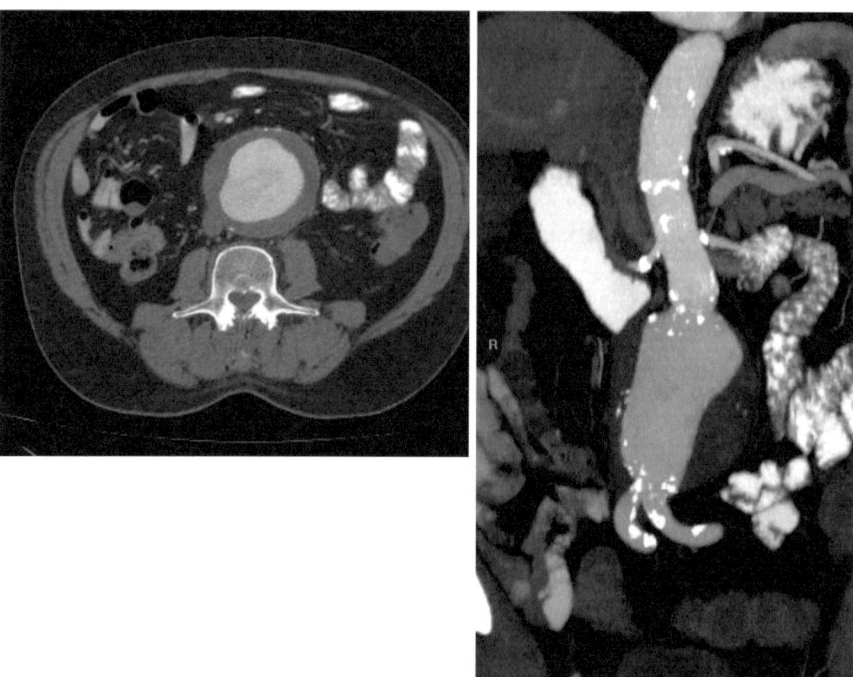

Fig. 25.1 CT scan of an 8 cm abdominal aneurysm in a 76-years old male

A 72-year-old patient with history of diabetes and hypertension, underwent to an abdominal ultrasound that revealed infrarenal abdominal aortic aneurysm. CT scan performed after few days confirmed the 8 cm fusiform infrarenal abdominal aneurysm (Fig. 25.1). The case was discussed in a multidisciplinary setting, and an endovascular treatment was scheduled.

The length and angle of proximal neck and the non-involvement of the iliac arteries was favorable for an infrarenal stent-graft (Fig. 25.2). This endoprosthesis can be considered because of the length and the angle of the proximal neck. The diameters and the lengths of the endograft were planned on the CT scan performed before the intervention, using MPR reconstruction (Fig. 25.3).

Procedure was performed in local anesthesia and mild sedation.

After preliminary angiogram the main body of the stent-graft was introduced through the right femoral access while the contralateral branch through the left common femoral artery (Fig. 25.4).

The aortic angiogram at the end of procedure showed correct position and complete exclusion of the aneurysm.

CT performed at 30 days showed complete exclusion of the aneurysm (Fig. 25.5).

Fig. 25.2 Commercially available infrarenal stent-graft in case of long and straight proximal neck (2–3 cm)

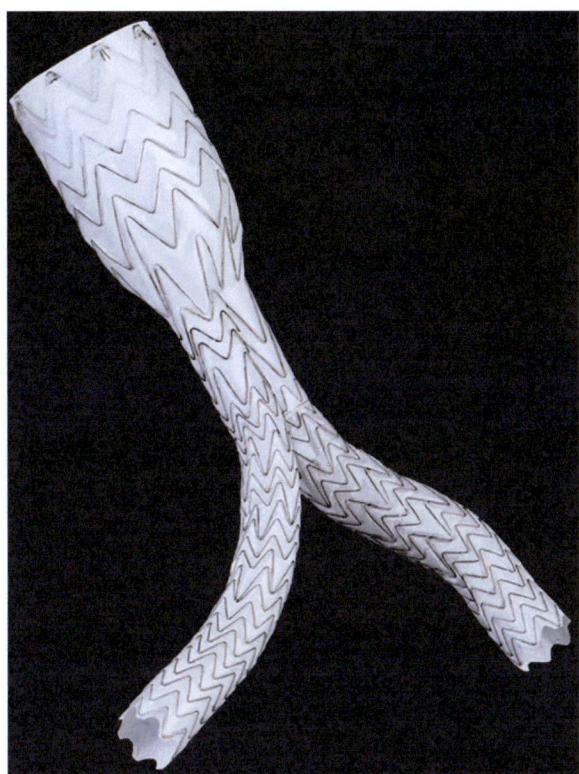

1. Finding suggests:
   (a) Infrarenal abdominal aneurysm with signs of rupture
   (b) Infrarenal abdominal aneurysm without evidence of rupture
   (c) Infrarenal abdominal aneurysm with iliac arteries involvement
   (d) Thoraco-abdominal aortic aneurysm
2. Which next step would you recommend to the patient?
   (a) US follow-up
   (b) CT or MRI follow-up
   (c) Multidisciplinary evaluation and treatment
   (d) Vascular screening
3. Which of the following is false:
   (a) Surgical treatment would have been more appropriate in this case
   (b) Infrarenal stent-graft is a good choice in this case
   (c) Common bilateral femoral access is mandatory for EVAR
4. Which of the following is correct:
   (a) Type 2 endoleak is often observed after EVAR but treatment is recommended in case of sac enlargement
   (b) Type 1 endoleak is commonly observed after EVAR and often no other treatments are necessary in case of sac stability

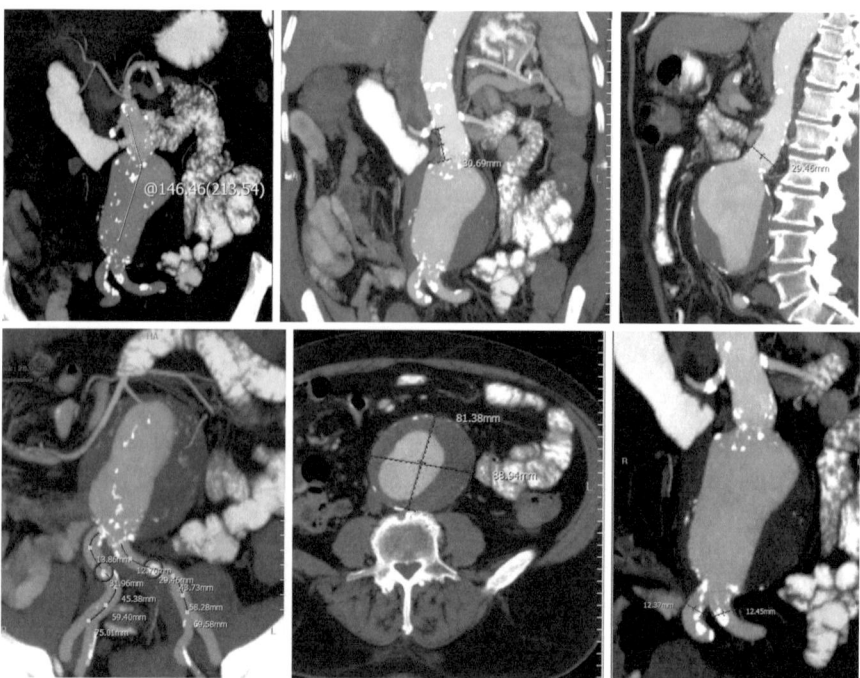

Fig. 25.3 MPR reconstructions performed to assess the parameters for correct sizing of the stent-graft

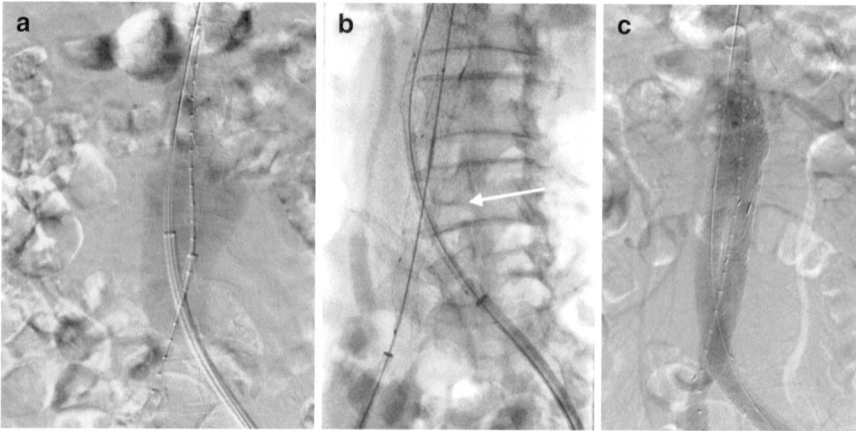

Fig. 25.4 Procedure: aortic angiogram confirming infrarenal aortic aneurysm (**a**). Iliac branches were deployed in twisted mode to avoid kinking of the iliac grafts, due to the narrow angle between iliac arteries and aorta (**b**). Final angiogram showed patency of the stent-graft (**c**)

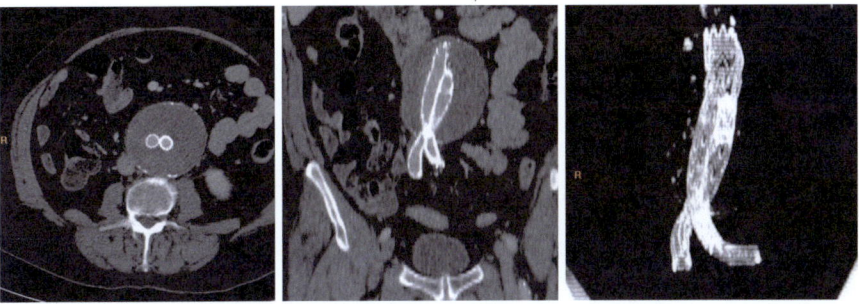

Fig. 25.5 CT scan performed 30 days after procedure

(c) Type 2 endoleak doesn't require treatment even if an increase of the aneurysm is observed
(d) Every type of endoleak is an emergency and requires treatment

Answers
1. (b)
2. (c)
3. (a)
4. (a)

Case 5

Simone CiagliaBianca Rocco, and Pier Giorgio Nardis

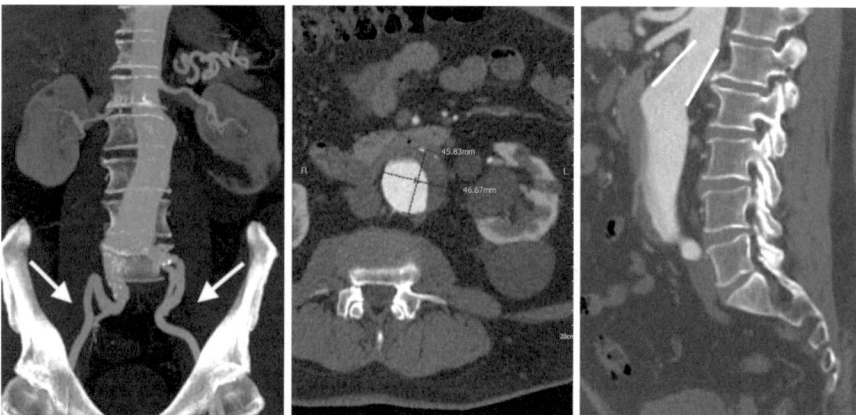

Fig. 25.6 CT scan of a juxtarenal abdominal aortic aneurysm with tapered neck and significant tortuosity of iliac arteries

A 64-year-old patient, with history of hypertension, followed up with ultrasound for a 3.8 cm abdominal aortic aneurysm showed rapid increase of the sac at last US follow-up.

CT scan performed after a week confirmed a 4.5 cm juxtarenal abdominal aortic aneurysm, with a short conic-shape proximal neck (Fig. 25.6). The case was discussed in a multidisciplinary team and an endovascular treatment was proposed. In consideration of the anatomy of the patient and the shape and length of the proximal neck, the endograft considered was a juxtarenal stent-graft. This endoprosthesis can be used also in case of short proximal neck thanks to its free flow element that can be positioned across the renal arteries (Fig. 25.7).

Also in this case, MPR reconstructions were useful to plan the diameters and the length of the endograft (Fig. 25.8).

The procedure was performed in local anesthesia and mild sedation.

Bilateral percutaneous common femoral artery access was performed. From the right femoral access, the main body and right iliac branch were introduced, while the left femoral access was used to introduce the left iliac branch.

Type II endoleak was observed due to a little downshift of the stent-graft; a short aortic cuff just below the renal arteries was released to achieve proximal sealing. The final angiogram showed patency and of the endografts with complete exclusion of the aneurysm (Fig. 25.9).

CT scan performed 30 days showed type II endoleak from lumbar arteries without sac enlargement; therefore, the patient was placed on follow-up without further interventions (Fig. 25.10).

Fig. 25.7 This endoprosthesis is indicated in case of short proximal neck. The free flow element permits a proximal ceiling at the level of renal arteries

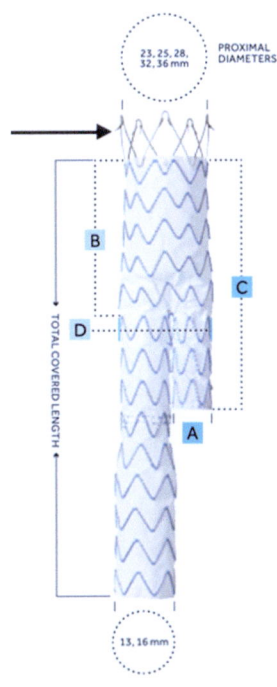

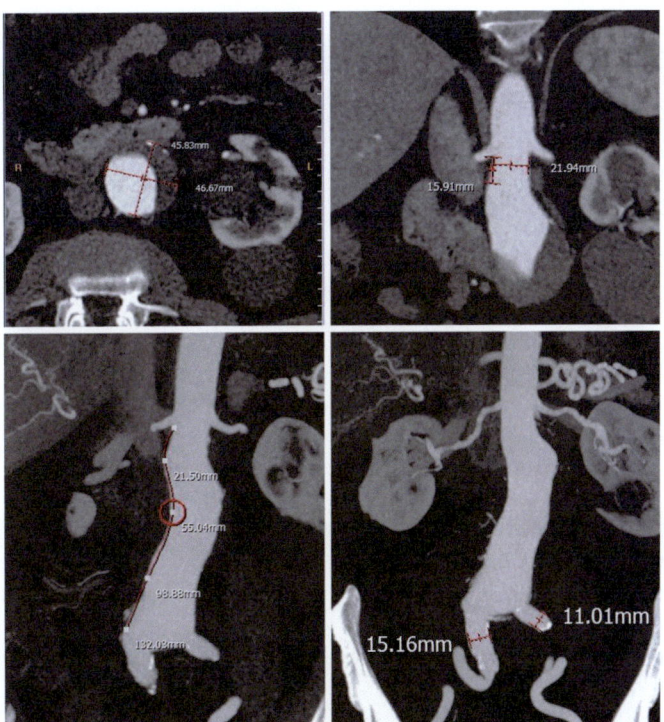

Fig. 25.8 MPR reconstructions used to assess the correct sizing of the endograft

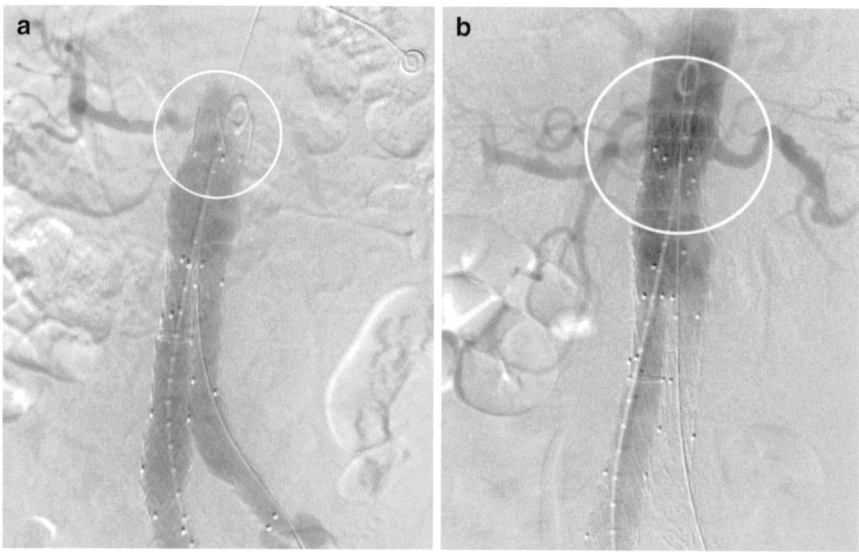

Fig. 25.9 Procedure: the angiogram performed after graft deployment showed a little downshift of the endoprosthesis. The proximal markers of the graft were not well aligned with renal arteries (**a**) so a cuff was positioned to achieve a good proximal ceiling. The final angiogram showed good position of the two grafts and no endoleak was observed (**b**)

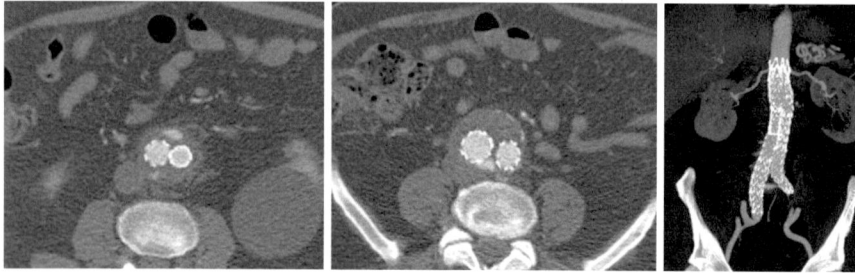

Fig. 25.10 CT scan performed after 30 days showed patency of the stent-graft; type II endoleak is commonly observed at early follow-up

1. What additional findings should be reported?
    (a) Severe dilatation of common iliac arteries
    (b) Tortuous iliac arteries and conical-shape of proximal neck
    (c) Signs of imminent rupture
    (d) Aneurysm involving renal arteries
2. Considering the shortness of proximal neck and its tapered-shape, which endoprosthesis would be better to choose?
    (a) An endoprosthesis with free flow component so can be released across renal arteries
    (b) An iliac branch endoprosthesis
    (c) An infrarenal endoprosthesis

(d) Surgical treatment is mandatory in this case
3. This procedure:
   (a) Requires just single common femoral access
   (b) Requires bilateral common femoral access
   (c) The iliac tortuosity was not a problem
   (d) It is often burdened with more complications compared to surgery
4. Which of the following is true:
   (a) CT scan after procedure is not required, just US follow-up is recommended
   (b) MRI follow-up could be a good alternative to CT scan
   (c) CEUS is the preferred follow-up in obese patient
   (d) CT scan must be performed according to the evidence of endoleak and aneurysm changing

Answers
1. (b)
2. (a)
3. (b)
4. (d)

Case 6

Davide Curione

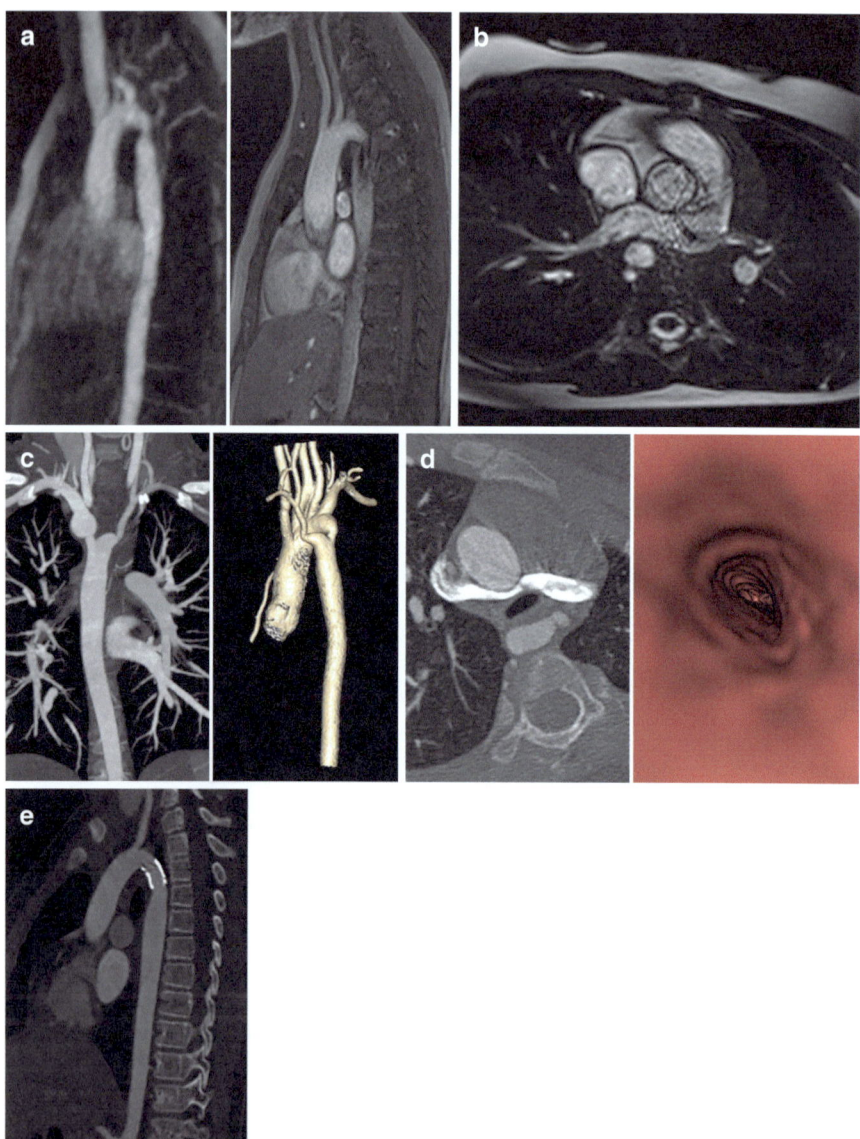

1. *Figure a shows*:
    (a) Aortic coarctation with flow acceleration at the isthmus
    (b) Aortic coarctation without collateral vessels

(c) Diffuse hypoplasia of the aortic arch without coarctation
(d) Right aortic arch with stenotic aberrant left subclavian artery
2. *The systolic cine image in Fig. b*:
   (a) Does not clearly define the morphology of the aortic valve due to artifacts
   (b) Demonstrates the association between aortic coarctation and bicuspid aortic valve
   (c) Displays a normal tricuspid aortic valve
   (d) Shows flow acceleration at the aortic isthmus
3. *In Fig. c there is*:
   (a) A post-stenotic aortic aneurysm distal to the site of coarctation
   (b) An aberrant right subclavian artery with Kommerell diverticulum proximal to the site of coarctation
   (c) An aberrant left subclavian artery without Kommerell diverticulum distal to the site of coarctation
   (d) A vascular ring due to right aortic arch and aberrant left subclavian artery with Kommerell diverticulum
4. *Figure d demonstrates*:
   (a) Tracheal stenosis caused by aortic coarctation
   (b) Tracheal stenosis caused by vascular ring
   (c) Tracheal stenosis caused by retroaortic left innominate vein
   (d) Tracheomalacia caused by all of the above-mentioned factors
5. *In Fig. e*:
   (a) Aortic coarctation underwent surgical treatment with patch calcification
   (b) Aortic coarctation underwent endovascular treatment with stent placement
   (c) Both aortic coarctation and vascular ring underwent treatment
   (d) Vascular ring underwent surgical treatment with resection of the ligamentum arteriosum
6. *Putting all the pieces together, which of the following statements is most likely true*:
   (a) The patient had atypical aortic coarctation and vascular ring but with typical clinical findings of upper extremity hypertension and dysphagia/dyspnea
   (b) The patient had typical aortic coarctation and vascular ring but with blood pressure drop in the left arm
   (c) The patient had hypertension only in the right arm
   (d) The patient certainly stopped having hypertension after being treated as is always the case in aortic coarctation

Answers
1. (a)
2. (c)
3. (d)
4. (b)
5. (b)
6. (c)

Case 7

Nunzia Di Meo

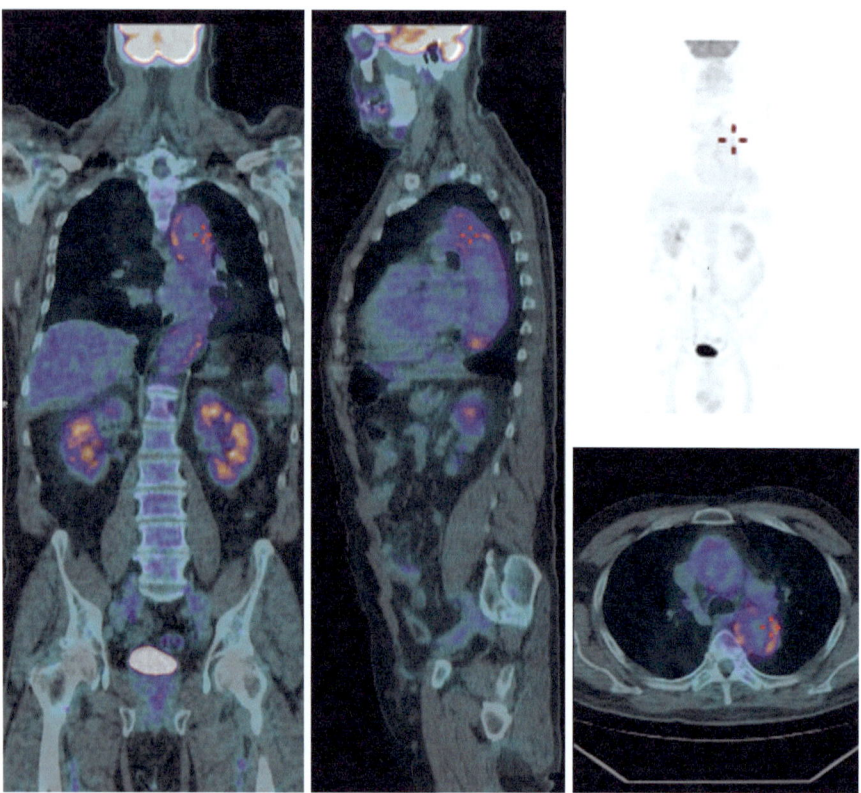

Fig. 25.11 PET-CT scan

A 70-year-old man, came to our observation, complaining a 1-month history of chest pain and increase of inflammatory markers (CRP 144 mg/L). The condition proved unresponsive to the medical treatment prescribed after a diagnosis of percarditis, made in a previous access to the Emergency Department. Lab test screening for infection, including viral serology, and for auto-antibody, including extractable-nuclear antigen and rheumatoid factor, were negative. Antineutrophil cytoplasmic antibody was positive. Echocardiogram showed no pericardial effusion and normal left ventricular function.

PET-CT (Fig. 25.11) and an MRI (Figs. 25.12 and 25.13) were performed.

25 Clinical Cases

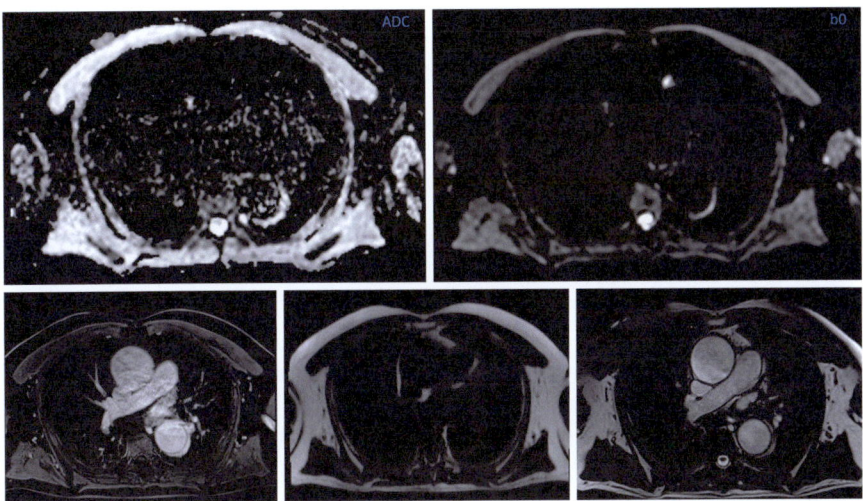

Fig. 25.12 MRI scan. Upper row: DWI, ADC map and b0. Lower row: contrast-enhanced 3d GE T! with fat suppression, T1/T2 black blood, and balanced T2

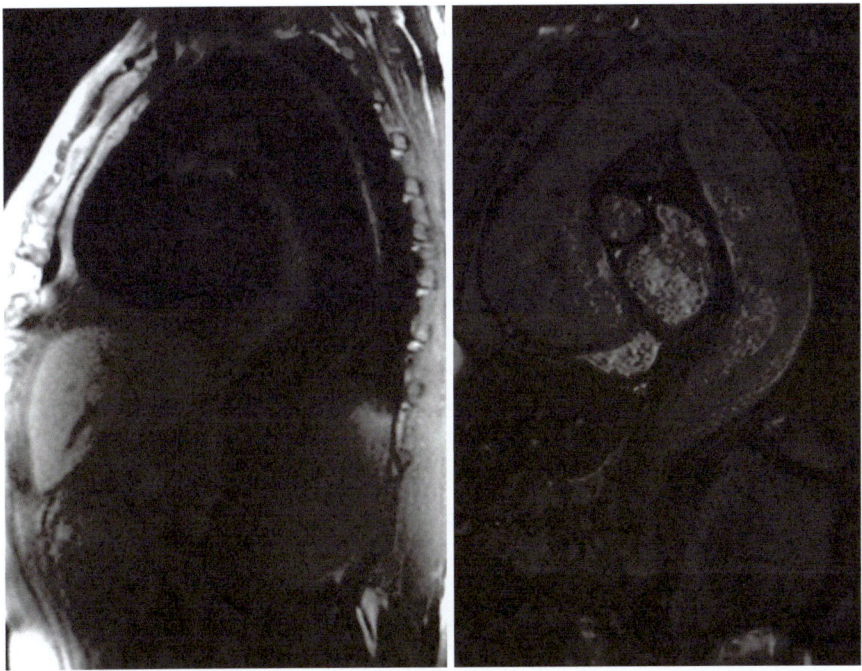

Fig. 25.13 MRI scan 3d SE T1 and 3d T2

1. Findings suggest:
   (a) Ascending aortic aneurysm
   (b) Intramural hematoma
   (c) Giant cell aortitis
   (d) 1 + 3
2. What ids the most common form of aortitis:
   (a) Infectious aortitis
   (b) Giant cell aortitis
   (c) Takayasu
   (d) Chronic periaortitis
3. Which of the following is false:
   (a) CTA has high spatial resolution and can help in the differential diagnosis between inflammatory disease and IMH
   (b) PET-CT has a good sensitivity and excellent specificity
   (c) MRI is superior to PET-CT and CTA, due to better contrast resolution
   (d) Ultrasound can show the halo sign in giant cell aortitis
4. What does the halo sign point at:
   (a) Impending rupture
   (b) Aneurysm
   (c) Aortic dissection
   (d) Parietal edema

Answers
1. (d)
2. (b)
3. (b)
4. (d)

Case 8

Teresa Falcone

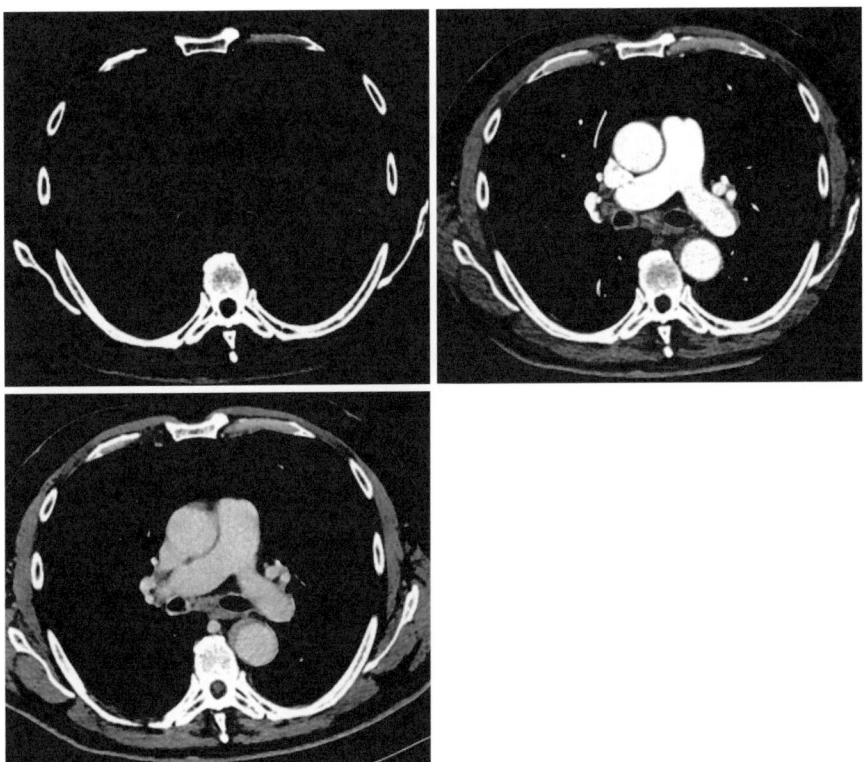

Fig. 25.14 CT scan. Axial unhanced, arterial, and venous phase

A 70-year-old male admitted to the hospital for chest pain of recent onset. The pain is described as moderate and radiating to the interscapular region. The patient is under treatment for hypertension. CT scan is performed (Fig. 25.14).

1. CT findings are consistent with:
    (a) Penetrating atherosclerotic ulcer (PAU)
    (b) Intramural hematoma (IMH)
    (c) Aortic atherosclerosis
    (d) Aortic dissection
2. In the present scenario, the most informative images are:
    (a) First pass CTA acquisition
    (b) Venous phase acquisition
    (c) Unenhanced acquisition
    (d) MIP reconstructions

3. In the present scenario, is ECG gating mandatory?
   (a) Yes, pulsation artifacts may significantly degrade image quality
   (b) No, unless the pathology involves the ascending aorta
   (c) No, it can be replaced by high-pitch ungated acquisition, depending on the heart rate
   (d) No, unless the aortic aneurysm is >35 mm
4. Which of the above is wrong?
   (a) Crescent-shape hyperattenuation (>50 HU) of the aortic wall suggest IMH
   (b) Bulging of the external aortic contour suggests PAU
   (c) Intimal tear suggests aortic dissection
   (d) Spiral longitudinal progression suggests IMH

Answers
1. (b)
2. (c)
3. (b)
4. (d)

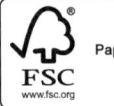

If you have any concerns about our products,
you can contact us on
ProductSafety@springernature.com

In case Publisher is established outside the EU,
the EU authorized representative is:
**Springer Nature Customer Service Center GmbH
Europaplatz 3, 69115 Heidelberg, Germany**

Printed by Libri Plureos GmbH
in Hamburg, Germany